The Kidneys

The Kidneys

Balancing the Fluids

TORSTAR BOOKS
New York • Toronto

TORSTAR BOOKS INC.
41 Madison Avenue, Suite 2900
New York, NY 10010

THE HUMAN BODY
The Kidneys:
Balancing the Fluids

Publisher
Bruce Marshall

Art Editor:
John Bigg

Creation Coordinator
Harold Bull

Editor:
John Clark

Managing Editor
Ruth Binney

Commissioning Editor
Hal Robinson

Contributors
Arthur Boylston, Loraine Fergusson,
Angela Garner, Paulette Pratt, Saffron
Whitehead

Text Editors
Wendy Allen, Lloyd Lindo, Maria Pal

Researchers
Angela Bone, Jazz Wilson

Picture Researchers
Jan Croot, Dee Robinson

Layout and Visualization
Ted McCausland, Rita Wuthrich

Artists
Mick Gillah, Aziz Khan, Mick
Saunders, Shirley Willis

Cover Design
Moonink Communications

Cover Art
Paul Giovanopoulos

Production Director
Barry Baker

Production Coordinator
Janice Storr

Business Coordinator
Candy Lee

Planning Assistant
Avril Essery

International Sales
Barbara Anderson

In conjunction with this series Torstar Books offers an electronic digital thermometer which provides accurate body temperature readings in large liquid crystal numbers within 60 seconds.

For more information write to:
Torstar Books Inc.
41 Madison Avenue, Suite 2900
New York, NY 10010

Marshall Editions, an editorial group that specializes in the design and publication of scientific subjects for the general reader, prepared this book. Marshall has written and illustrated standard works on technology, animal behavior, computer usage and the tropical rain forests which are recommended for schools and libraries as well as for popular reference.

Series Consultants

Donald M. Engelman is Professor of Molecular Biophysics and Biochemistry and Professor of Biology at Yale. He has pioneered new methods for understanding cell membranes and ribosomes, and has also worked on the problem of atherosclerosis. He has published widely in professional and lay journals and lectured at many universities and international conferences. He is also involved with National Advisory Groups concerned with Molecular Biology, Cancer, and the operation of National Laboratory Facilities.

Stanley Joel Reiser is Professor of Humanities and Technology in Health Care Center in Houston. He is the author of *Medicine and the Reign of Technology* , coeditor of *Ethics in Medicine: Historical Perspectives and Contemporary Concerns*, and coeditor of the anthology *The Machine at the Bedside*.

Harold C. Slavkin, Professor of Biochemistry at the University of Southern California, directs the Graduate Program in

Craniofacial Biology and also serves as Chief of the Laboratory for Developmental Biology in the University's Gerontology Center. His research on the genetic basis of congenital defects of the head and neck has been widely published.

Lewis Thomas is Chancellor of the Memorial Sloan-Kettering Cancer Center in New York City and University Professor at the State University of New York, Stony Brook. A member of the National Academy of Sciences, Dr. Thomas has served on advisory councils of the National Institutes of Health.

Consultants *for* The Kidneys

Thomas McGovern is a practicing physician specializing in urology and a member of the Admissions Committee at Cornell University Medical College. His papers and other publications include results of studies on the use of ultrasonography in urological investigations.

Robert S. Waldbaum is a Clinical Associate Professor of Surgery (Urology) at the Cornell University Medical College and Director of Urology at the North Shore University Hospital. He is a fellow of the American College of Surgeons, the International Society of Urology and the Society for Pediatric Urology. After a college major in vertebrate zoology and paleontology, he remains an avid amateur biologist.

Medical Advisor
Arthur Boylston

Library of Congress
Cataloging in Publication Data

Main entry under title:

The Kidneys: Balancing the Fluids

   Includes index.
   1. Kidneys.   2. Nephrology–popular works.
3. Kidneys–diseases–popular works.
I. Torstar books (firm)
[DNLM: 1. Kidney–physiology–popular works.
WJ 301 K464]
QP249.K54   1986   612'.463   86-1914

ISBN 0-920269-22-2 (The Human Body Series)
ISBN 0-920269-21-4 (The Kidneys)
ISBN 1-55001-000-x (leatherbound)
ISBN 0-920269-96-6 (school ed.)

20 19 18 17 16 15 14 13 12 11
10   9   8   7   6   5   4   3   2   1

Printed in Belgium

Contents

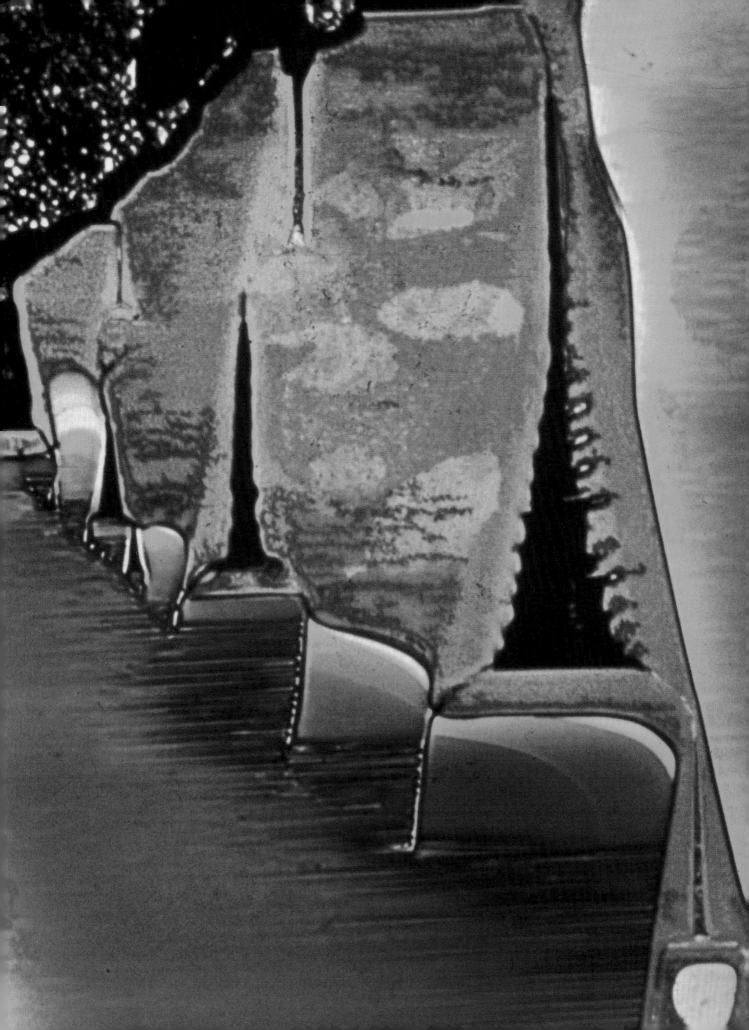

Introduction:

Maintaining the Internal Environment

The way some people describe the human body, it might be thought that inside it there are some bones, a few organs, one or two other bits and pieces, and all are floating in a vast sea of internal fluids. Yet that is not as ludicrously exaggerated as it may sound. The body is, after all, more than two-thirds liquid in overall volume. Of course it is not just one sort of liquid — blood is obviously the major form, but there are others, some as vital. Almost all have one constituent in common: water. Even blood plasma is ninety per cent water. So we all have to drink water in quantity.

In control of regulating most of the water in the body are the kidneys. Their main functions are to filter the blood of impurities, to drain off wastes, and to maintain the balance of essential chemicals in the body in liquid form. All these functions are carried out by the same single process.

The filtration is complex but extremely practical, performed through myriad tiny capillaries in the renal medulla. It is this operation that is the central element of the dialysis machine, the "artificial kidney." Draining off wastes produces urine, ducted through the ureter from each kidney to the bladder, and passed out from there through the urethra. In former times, stones (calculi) used to be common — and occasionally dangerous — in the bladder; dietary changes have since then made them considerably rarer. The maintenance of the correct balance of fluids in the body is a function that is at least as important as either of the other two. It is not merely a question of allowing more urine to be made if we drink more than normal; but one also of regulating the amount and comparative strengths of various salts in solution, of lubricating certain tissues and servicing some glands (such as the sweat glands); above all, the blood has to be kept clean so that the whole body — which depends on it for nutrients and the transportation of hormones and essential elements — continues to function optimally.

Uric acid, shown here crystallized on a microscope slide, is normally secreted in the urine in the form of urate salts. But if the kidneys do not function properly, the urate concentration in the blood increases and the substance may accumulate in the joints of the hands and feet, causing gout. In most patients, this painful disorder is of genetic origin.

7

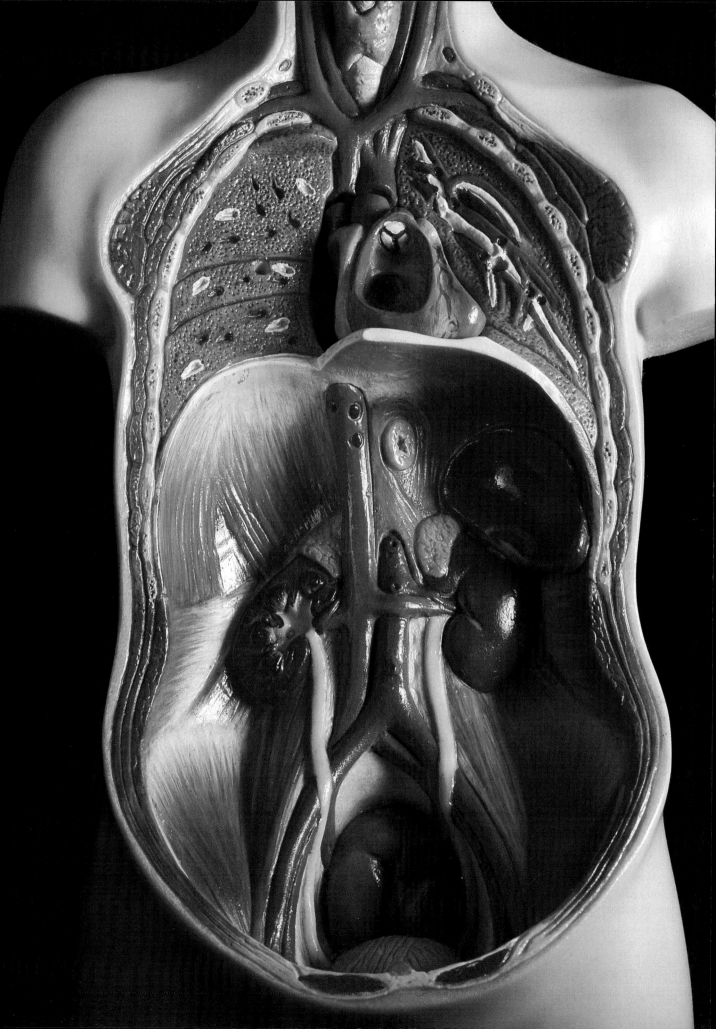

Chapter 1

The Water of Life

When we contemplate physical well-being, we tend to think only of input — getting enough oxygen, food and fluids — rather than of the somewhat less appealing business of waste disposal. In terms of body maintenance, however, excretion is just as essential as breathing air and eating food. For, just like any processing plant taking in raw materials, using them, and turning out the waste materials unused or left over, the human body has a continuing need to rid itself of wastes. If it could not shed the chemical wastes which are by-products of metabolism, these unwanted substances — most of them toxic to some extent — would begin to accumulate in the tissues, causing metabolic disturbances, illness and, finally, death.

Exit routes through which these wastes can be eliminated include the skin, the lungs (in the case of carbon dioxide and water vapor) and the intestines. But the principal organs of excretion are the kidneys, which process excess water, mineral salts and most of the urea (which is a nitrogen-containing breakdown product of protein metabolism). The kidneys are paired organs which receive blood from the renal arteries leading off the main aorta, and are drained by the renal veins. All the blood in the circulation passes through the kidneys almost twenty times in an hour, with about one-fifth of its volume being filtered at each circuit.

The active sites of filtration are the glomeruli — about a million to each kidney — each consisting of a sphere of coiled blood vessels cupped in a fine-walled sac (Bowman's capsule). Blood enters the glomeruli under pressure and about one-fifth of its plasma is forced through the capillary walls, which are permeable to small molecules of waste, including some proteins, but hold back large protein molecules and the red and white cells and platelets of the blood. Most of the water and useful substances are reabsorbed into the blood. The remainder of the filtrate is processed as urine and carried away in the ureters. These lead away from

The human body is nearly two-thirds water. That its survival on any level is possible depends to a large degree on the functions and processes performed by the kidneys. The vital control of the kidney's management of salt and water on which terrestrial life depends consists of a series of interactions between the kidney itself, the brain and pituitary gland, blood vessels and the adrenal glands. Between them the volume and composition of the body fluids is kept in balance.

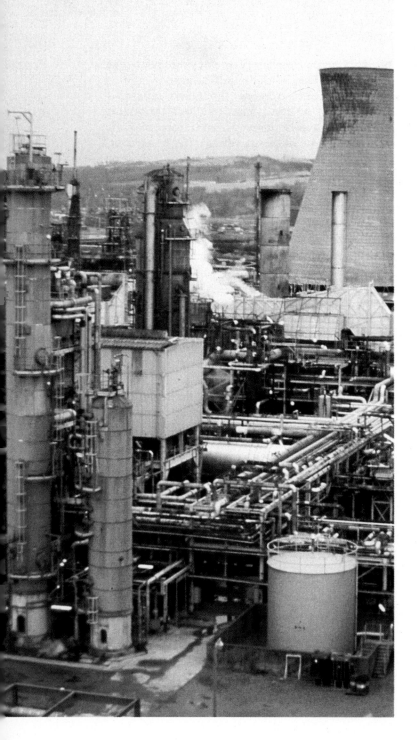

Like a miniature chemical processing plant, the kidneys control the quantity and destination of all fluid inputs and various minerals derived from food, conserving what is needed and disposing of the wastes.

the inner pelvis of the kidney and from them the filtrate is passed to the bladder and, from this muscular reservoir, voided by way of the urethra.

Some of the fluid is retained, however, for the kidneys are not concerned merely with "cleansing" the blood, they are involved also with fluid conservation. Unlike aquatic creatures, in which kidneys evolved as simple organs of excretion to get rid of water excess, air-breathing land-based vertebrates, including humans, are at constant risk from water-depletion. If all the fluid filtered off in the kidneys of a human were converted to urine, that person would become severely dehydrated within an hour. So the renal tubules are also instrumental in recycling: transferring water, salts and sugars back through their membranous walls to be returned to the bloodstream. Following reabsorption, all that remains in the nephrons is a concentrated solution of waste — mainly urea — which, mixed with secretions from the kidney itself, forms the urine.

The kidneys also exercise selective control over the retention or release of mineral salts. The balance of sodium and potassium is regulated by adrenal hormones (the corticosteroids), and the secretions of the parathyroid glands influence levels of phosphate and calcium. By fulfilling an active role in such transactions, the kidneys make a vital contribution to the condition of homeostasis (the internal equilibrium of the body as a whole). If these small but infinitely complex organs ever lose their facility of action, the correct balance and composition of body fluids is rapidly disturbed.

The Sieve and Filtration

Only a hundred years ago one physician complained that "All we know *for certain* about the kidney is that it makes urine." That the kidneys are part of the urinary system has been recognized since the time of Aristotle, if not earlier. Galen, the Roman physician of the second century A.D., whose theories were to persist for more than a thousand years, suggested that the interior of the kidney was a sieve which filtered out impurities into the urine. Even Vesalius, the great sixteenth-century anatomist of Brussels, could not free himself from Galen's influence: he showed the kidney with its "sieve." Real breakthroughs in

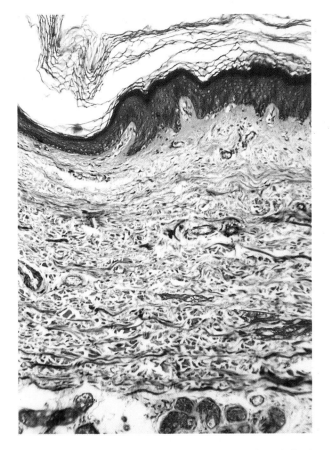

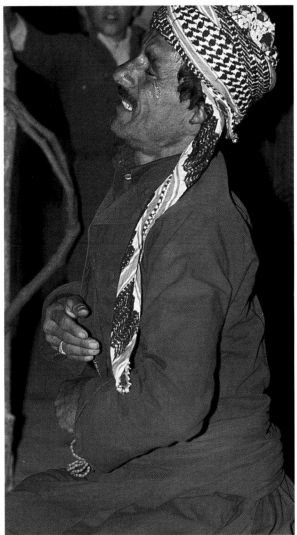

knowledge of the kidney had to await the skilled microscopists of later centuries.

Unlike that of the heart or intestines, the gross anatomy of the kidney reveals almost nothing of its finer workings. The men who first observed the nephron and its contents were thus quite incapable of interpreting their discoveries. The Italian anatomist Marcello Malpighi turned his microscope on renal tissue and published his findings on the glomerulus (the "little ball" of the kidney) in 1659. But in challenging Galen's mythical sieve he outraged his colleagues, who denounced him and even set upon him.

Long after Malpighi had been battered for his insights, the English physician William Bowman wrote the treatise which was to prove a watershed in renal studies: "On the Structure and Use of the Malpighian Bodies of the Kidney with Observations on the Circulation through that Gland" (1842). Although he described accurately how

water and wastes were filtered out of the glomerulus and into the tubule, he failed to realize that the tubules were also engaged in the reabsorption and secretion of water and salts. Only two years later, Carl Ludwig, working in Vienna, published his findings on renal physiology. Ludwig declared that the rate of filtration through the glomerulus depended on the blood pressure, and that the filtrate was concentrated in the tubules. Building on Ludwig's work, a Scottish Professor of Pharmacology, A. R. Cushny, finally set out in detail the filtration-reabsorption theory during World War I in 1917.

Today renal function is evaluated by what is called the glomerular filtration rate (GFR): the amount of a substance cleared from the blood in one minute. The possibility of using the kidney's filtering activity in this way was suggested by the American physiologist Homer Smith in 1965. "In my opinion," he wrote, "this word [clearance] has

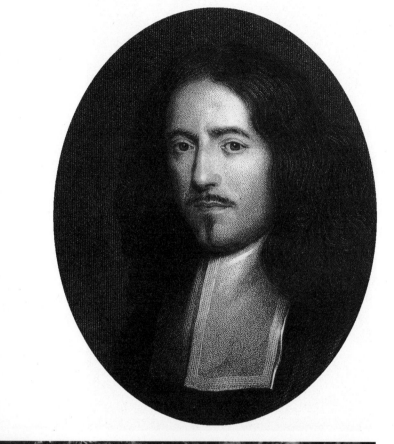

Through microscopic anatomy, Malpighi discovered structures previously unaccounted for. One was the glomerulus (bottom), the key regulator of blood-processing in the kidney.

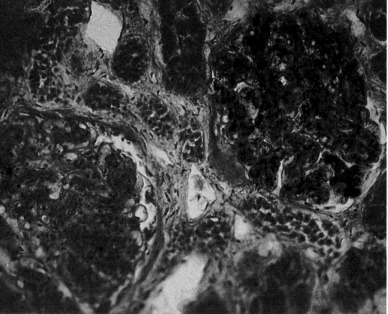

been more useful to renal physiology than all the equations ever written.''

Early Diagnosis of Kidney Disorders

The caduceus — the staff of the messenger-god Mercury — is widely recognized as a symbol of modern medical services. It was preceded, however, by a far more unlikely symbol — the uroscope. In medieval or Renaissance art, a physician may always be identified by the bottle of urine he holds up for examination. The ubiquitous uroscope gives us some inkling of the significance attached to the appearance of urine in diagnosis.

Salerno in southern Italy became a center of medical learning in the ninth century, drawing teachers from among Christian, Jewish and Arab physicians. Its chief contribution to uroscopy came from the teachings of the early medieval master Isaac Judaeus, from whose time urine became a favorite theme for treatises and learned discourse. Color, odor and the formation of sediment were all studied assiduously; and the differing layers within the urine in a glass beaker were believed to correspond to the different regions of the body.

Eventually, throughout Europe, this absurd practice displaced examination of the patient. The sight of an assistant hurrying through the streets, little wicker basket in hand, to bring a ''sample'' to the physician from the bedside was commonplace. In the sixteenth century, the Royal College of Physicians in London registered its disapproval by forbidding treatment based only on uroscopy.

Nevertheless, uroscopy had its origins in sound clinical observation. By the fifth century B.C. the Hippocratic school had already recognized that certain characteristic changes in the urine were dignostic of kidney or bladder conditions. Blood or pus indicated infection; bubbles on the surface meant kidney failure; spontaneous appearance of blood pointed to hemorrhage in the kidney, and sandy sediment was indicative of a stone. Aulus Cornelius Celsus — a Roman nobleman of the first century B.C. — also associated frequent, copious urine and pain in the kidney region with kidney disease. It was the gradual erosion of this fund of Classical knowledge that debased what had once been a sound practice to a meaningless ritual.

Eventually, the study of urine led back to the

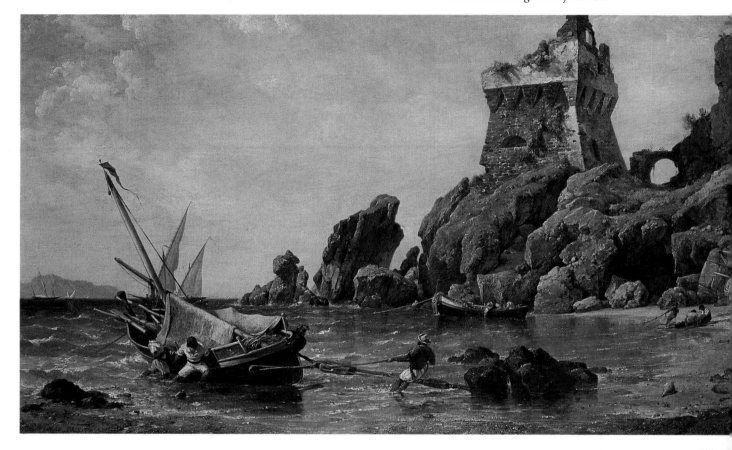

study of the kidneys. While making his traditional examination of urine, Frederick Dekkers of Leyden (1648–1720) observed that some specimens of urine coagulated when heated. This singular phenomenon was picked up by Domenico Cotugno of Naples, who recalled that fluid drawn from patients with dropsy, or edema (a condition in which serous fluid accumulates in cellular tissue or in a body cavity), also coagulated. He repeated Dekkers' experiment on a grand scale, heating two pints of urine and, in 1765, reported seeing "a white mass, already loosely coagulated like egg albumin." At the same time, Rosen von Rosenstein, working in Uppsala, Sweden, made the connection between scarlet fever and the presence of blood in the urine.

By the 1770s, the chemical composition of urine was being analyzed, and urea was identified as the primary waste product from the metabolism of protein. In 1776, the Swedish chemist Carl Wilhelm Scheele also separated out uric acid, which was subsequently implicated in gout. By 1827, London physician Richard Bright was able to state: "I have never yet examined the body of a patient dying with dropsy attended with coagulable urine, in whom some obvious derangement was not discovered in the kidneys." Modern nephrology was finally catching up with the physicians of the late Roman Empire who had associated dropsy with advanced renal disease and who related changes in urine to disorders of the excretory system.

The coagulation test, which crudely identified the presence of excess protein in the urine, offered the first diagnostic procedure for nephritis. "When the albumin is proved to exist, however slight . . . I look upon it with anxiety," wrote Bright. His observations of patients who were wasting away, both during their prolonged illness and *post mortem*, enabled him to define renal failure: "What appears to be the great office of the kidney — the

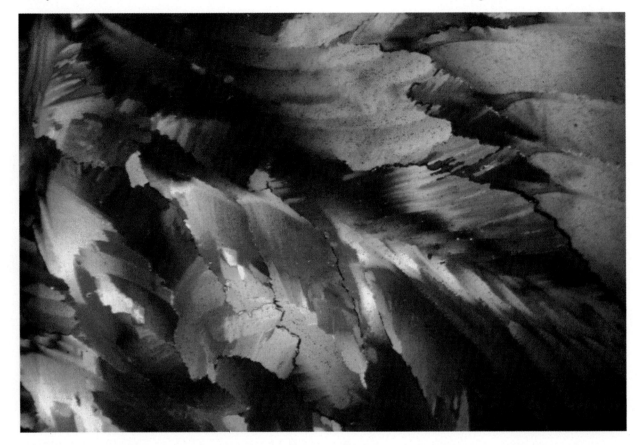

depuration of the blood — does not take place.''

Thanks to the mechanical ingenuity of another English doctor, Frederick Mahomed (1849–1884), it became possible to measure arterial blood pressure. Bright had noted a full, hard pulse in his patients and found damage to the heart and pericardium at autopsy; now hypertension was associated with kidney failure. Subsequent studies of patients with Bright's disease (a type of glomerulonephritis) revealed that several conditions could produce the same final pathway. The introduction of renal biopsy — taking samples of live tissue — was the key to differentiating between these disorders, enabling doctors to treat their patients before the kidneys suffered irreparable damage.

Treatments for "the Stone"

Meanwhile, physicians and surgeons had been treating diseases of the urinary system long before there was any understanding of the structure or function of the organs and tissues involved. In relation to the kidney, diagnosis outstripped treatment. Renal failure was recognized in the Hippocratic *Aphorisms*, but alleviation of symptoms stretched only as far as bleedings, diuretics, aperients and an assortment of repellent potions containing ingredients such as ox-dung and copper. Some bladder disorders were obvious from the inability to pass urine (retention). Because this problem was basically one of "mechanics," it was more accessible to treatment than other conditions —if the cause of the blockage could be found.

Most often urinary retention was caused by bladder stones (vesical calculi). Benjamin Franklin — who had to travel to the Constitutional Convention in a sedan chair because of the pain of his stone — wrote a classic description of the symptoms. He was more comfortable with a full bladder; he experienced spasmodic pain, interrupted flow of urine and blood in the urine. Declining

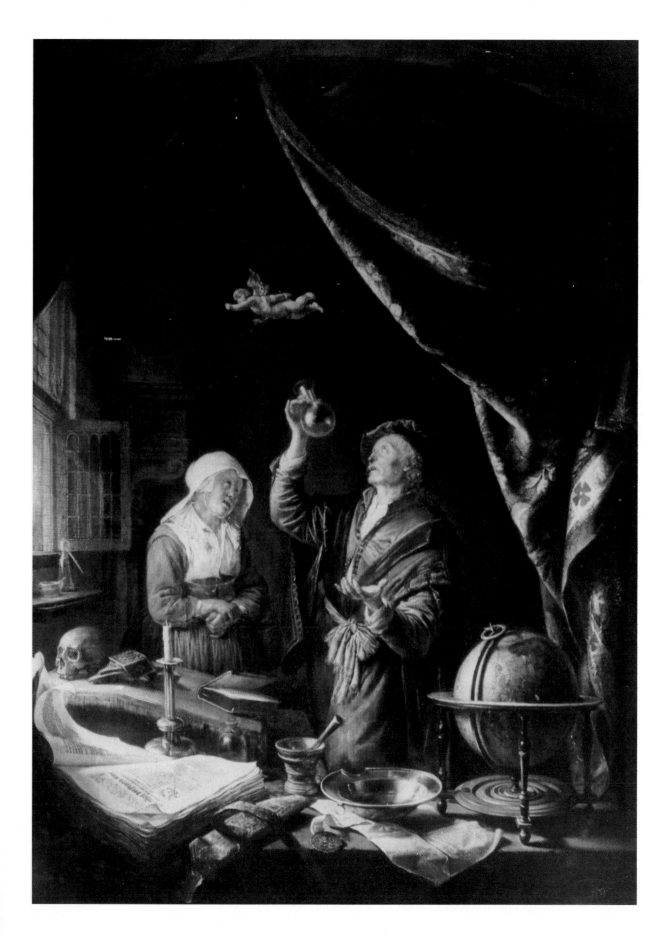

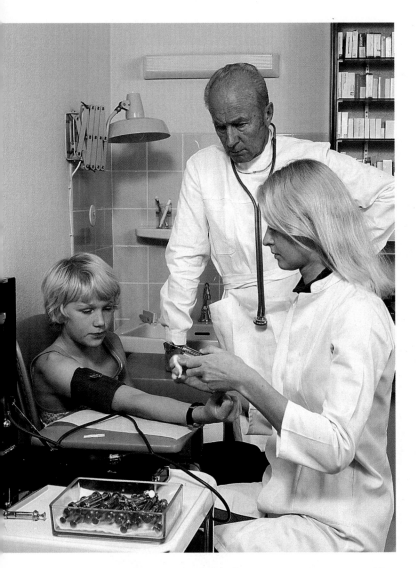

to submit to the knife, he spent the last years of his life in bed, reduced to a "skeleton covered by skin." Franklin was not unique. Both the English diarist Samuel Pepys in 1658 and American Chief Justice John Marshall in 1831 put themselves in the hands of lithotomists.

The art of "cutting for stone" — lithotomy — has a long history, distinct from the rest of urology. Even before the anatomy of the pelvic organs was known, bladder calculi were more amenable to surgery than most other complaints. The pain and inability to pass urine were directly attributable to stones in the bladder, the distention of which could be felt when the abdomen was palpated (examined by hand pressure). Removal of the stones often relieved both symptoms. The suffering of the patients can perhaps be better appreciated when it is realized that each voluntarily took the risk of trusting to the hands of a lithotomist who could not offer the benefits of aseptic technique and

anesthesia, and who in any case may well have been a charlatan.

Vesical calculi, today uncommon in the developed world, were once so common that kings appointed their own court lithotomists; and the stones removed in nineteenth-century London were said to be numerous enough to pave a road. The precise etiology of these obstructive rocks is unknown, but most were probably secondary to some form of obstruction or caused by poor diet. Physicians since Hippocrates' day held themselves aloof from the risky, messy business of lithotomy. Persons who performed it generally limited their practice to this one specialty; indeed, Duke Stanislas of Lorraine set up a school for lithotomists in the eighteenth century. Other operators served an apprenticeship with the master lithotomist or — much less satisfactorily — with itinerant practitioners. Such was the preoccupation with stones that in 1739 the British Parliament voted to pay Joanna Stephens the sum of £5,000 to disclose the formula of her stone-dissolving potion, a concoction of powdered snails and eggshell, infused herbs and burnt seed, rosehip and soap.

Apart from Hippocrates' proscription — he forbade physicians to cut for stones — the first outstanding mention of lithotomy occurs in the writings of Celsus. A professional dilettante who obviously had gained a sound knowledge of anatomy and of surgical procedures, he wrote a lucid description of perineal lithotomy, although it is not known whether he performed it himself. The procedure appeared again in the writings of Ambroise Paré, the brilliant self-taught barber-surgeon who attended the French court in the sixteenth century. Having learned his trade in military service, Paré preferred experience to theory when it came to operating technique, but apparently even he did not stoop to practice.

Arguably the greatest lithotomist of all time — and many practitioners attracted a following — was Pierre Franco, who probably learned his trade from an itinerant stone-cutter. His treatises, published in France in 1556 and 1561, not only bore the marks of an experienced practitioner, they also anticipated the major developments which rendered perineal lithotomy (using an incision in the crotch) far less hazardous. Moreover, Franco's

Symptoms of impending kidney disease are often deceptively mild in comparison to the potential severity of the disorder. The most observable symptoms of kidney malfunction are abnormalities in the volume, frequency and appearance of the urine. Other possible symptoms are swelling of the face and ankles, and pain in the upper back. Persistent feelings of tiredness, blurred vision or nausea occur in more serious renal disorders. A number of kidney diseases, including chronic pyelonephritis, glomerulonephritis, and kidney stones may, especially if left untreated, lead ultimately to kidney failure.

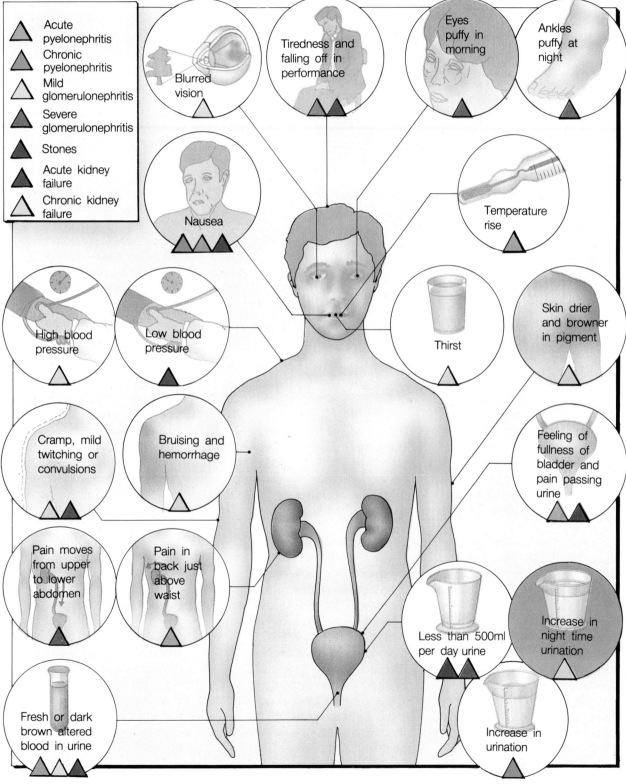

Acute pyelonephritis

Chronic pyelonephritis

Mild glomerulonephritis

Severe glomerulonephritis

Stones

Acute kidney failure

Chronic kidney failure

Blurred vision

Tiredness and falling off in performance

Eyes puffy in morning

Ankles puffy at night

Nausea

Temperature rise

High blood pressure

Low blood pressure

Thirst

Skin drier and browner in pigment

Cramp, mild twitching or convulsions

Bruising and hemorrhage

Feeling of fullness of bladder and pain passing urine

Pain moves from upper to lower abdomen

Pain in back just above waist

Less than 500ml per day urine

Increase in night time urination

Fresh or dark brown altered blood in urine

Increase in urination

Richard Bright

Clinical Observer

Holding a teaspoon over a candle flame, Richard Bright gently heated a sample of urine to reveal the presence of albumin—which established the link between edema and structural changes in the kidney. The term Bright's disease is now used to describe several conditions which produce similar symptoms, but his rudimentary experiment opened the way for the increasingly sophisticated treatment of kidney disorders.

One of the "great men of Guy's Hospital" in London during the first third of the nineteenth century, when that institution enjoyed an unrivaled reputation for the standard of its teaching, Bright's unique talent was for synthesis. Working closely with chemists, he pioneered the use of biochemical studies in diagnosis, which he coupled with meticulous observations.

Despite his unassuming character, Bright had a colorful early career. Born into a wealthy Bristol family in 1789, he enrolled at Edinburgh University in 1809 only to break off his medical studies to visit Iceland with Sir George Mackenzie. The trip spawned a life-long interest in zoology and botany and whetted Bright's appetite for travel. He packed his bags once again in 1814, a year after the

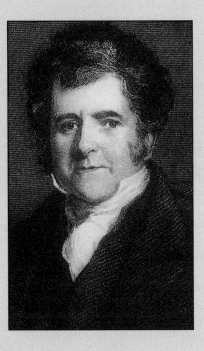

completion of his degree, reaching Brussels two weeks after the Battle of Waterloo.

His experiences working in European hospitals are recounted alongside his thoughts on art and politics in what many consider to be one of the finest travel books produced that century.

He returned to work at the London Fever Hospital, an act which almost cost him his life when he contracted a virus. Convalescence and another continental tour intervened before his appointment as Assistant Physician at Guy's in 1820. He was made Full Physician in 1824, a position he held until his death in 1858.

Bright contributed much to the teaching methods at Guy's, instilling in his students a sense of the importance of detailed observation and of establishing a close professional relationship with patients. Special clinical wards reserved for the study of specific diseases were another of his innovations.

His initial findings on kidney disorders were published in 1827, quickly establishing his reputation in that field. His researches covered a much wider area, however, encompassing the entire spectrum of internal medicine. With Thomas Addison he gave the first accurate description of appendicitis, and produced significant work on abdominal tumors, the brain and the nervous system.

In 1832 he was given the rare distinction of being elected Fellow of the Royal College of Physicians and, five years later, was made Physician Extraordinary to Queen Victoria.

Once questioned about his work, Bright would say only that he had brought "such facts together as seem to throw light upon each other"—playing down, with typical modesty, achievements that illuminated the many dark corners in medical knowledge that he explored.

account of the suprapubic lithotomy (using an incision in the lower abdomen — the approach now preferred) was the first description of this technique.

The classic perineal lithotomy, as set out by Franco, was performed on an unanesthetised patient, without any antiseptic regimen. While the sufferer was restrained in a semi-recumbent position, the lithotomist first inserted into the urethra a dilating instrument known as a sound, to feel for the stone and to try to bring it to the lowest point of the bladder. Then the assistant held the sound while the operator inserted two fingers of one hand into the rectum, using the other hand to make an incision at the base of the scrotum, cutting up through the prostate and into the bladder. The fingers in the rectum helped to locate the stone, for the wound was only large enough to feel for it. No attempt was made to work under direct vision.

Franco made two further recommendations — that the lithotomy be carried out in two stages, first the incision and second (some days later) removal of the stone; and that the wound be left open to heal. In later centuries, surgeons who chose to perform the full two-stage procedure enjoyed a success rate that would be acceptable today. It is now known that open wounds are more resistant to infection than closed wounds. The same fact underlines Franco's second precept — of open wound management. The secondary closure of contaminated wounds was finally adopted by field surgeons during World War I, when it was found that infection was less likely to develop. Franco's description of suprapubic lithotomy — which he did not recommend — and of the vastly increased risks encountered when the peritoneum was opened are indicative of an innovative, acutely observant and compassionate man.

Frère Jacques (of nursery-song fame) was a traveling lithotomist. Otherwise known as Jacques de Beaulieu, he served an apprenticeship and, adopting religious garb, took the road to Paris in 1697. Frère Jacques cut boldly, with a fine disregard for the rubrics of the resident lithotomists, plunging "his knife like a dagger into the perineum until it ground upon the stone." The disgruntled operators at the Hôtel-Dieu claimed that his stylish approach resulted in a mortality rate of more than

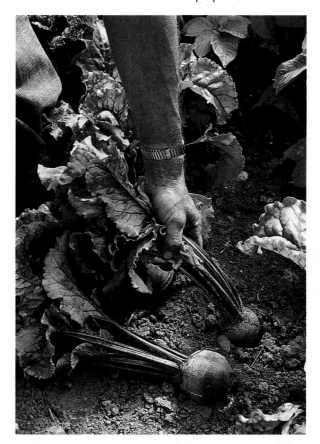

Occasionally the consumption of certain drugs or foods turns the urine a strange color. The best known of these is red beet which, because of it intense pigment, can turn the urine purple-red.

fifty per cent. The English observer William Lister claimed, however, that Jacques' rivals had falsified the statistics. Nobody will ever know; all that is certain is that the only real improvements in the survival rate came in the eighteenth century, with the advent of the professional lithotomists.

In the 1740s, Sauveur-François Morand traveled to London to observe the operating technique of William Cheselden at St Thomas's Hospital. At that time, lithotomy utilizing forceps was producing a mortality rate of forty-five per cent. Ironically, Cheselden, who did much to improve the professional standing of lithotomists, based his procedure on Franco's exposition and Frère Jacques' practice. One of Cheselden's greatest advances was a reduction in the time needed for the removal of the stone — from up to an hour to under a minute. His success rate, not even bettered at the beginning of the twentieth century, carried his fame across Europe.

This bizarre collection of minerals once lay within the confines of a human bladder. Unlike stones that form in the kidneys, bladder stones tend to be too large to pass naturally through the urethra and therefore have to be removed by surgical means. Although they vary in composition, most consist of concentric layers of one or more salts, including urates, calcium oxalate and phosphates.

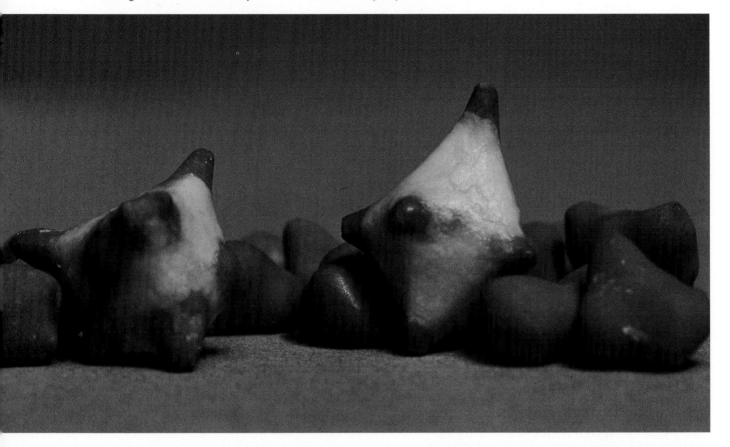

For those who enjoyed such things, the sixty-second lithotomy gained popularity as a public spectacle; the stone-cutter would make the cut and, at the moment of truth, brandish the extracted stone. It was short enough to hold the attention of the audience and ensure a quick succession of thrills. Frenchman Claude Pouteau, who also developed an obsession with cleanliness, denounced "the desire for instant glory which . . . has killed more patients than any other bad maneuver." Cutting with meticulous care, he lost only three patients in one hundred and twenty consecutive lithotomies.

The widespread acceptance of suprapubic lithotomy — access to the bladder via an incision made in the abdomen above the pubic bone — had to await the advent of asepsis and anesthetics. In 1881, Joseph Lister performed a perineal lithotomy, cleansing the wound with zinc chloride and leaving it open to heal. His patient made a good recovery.

The likelihood of penetrating the peritoneum of a conscious (and struggling) patient — and thus exposing the whole of the visceral cavity to infection — was dangerously real. Before Lister's time, surgeons accepted a mortality rate of more than 28 per cent following suprapubic lithotomy, mostly due to infection. Once Lister's principles, anticipated by Pouteau, were brought into use, the suprapubic approach rapidly replaced perineal lithotomy.

When having stones removed, women are decidedly favored by anatomy. In the female, the shortness of the urethra and its relative elasticity meant that lithotomists of old could reach the stones without having to cut for them. Rather than extract the calculi whole, operators introduced a crushing instrument which pulverized them and then removed the pieces — a technique termed lithotrity. The Greek surgeon Ammonius (c. 247 B.C.) employed this technique. The medieval Arabs developed a diamond-tipped probe to file away

20

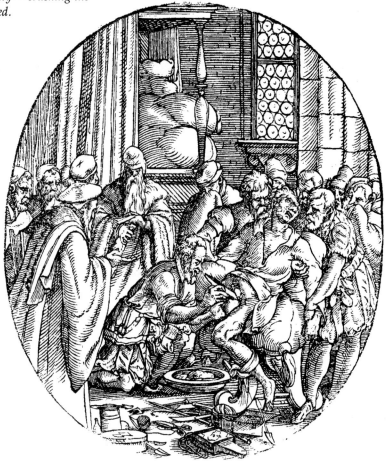

stone. But lithotrity began to be taken seriously only in the nineteenth century. Instruments incorporating a vise-like mechanism could exert a force of about four hundred pounds. The added refinement of suction irrigation was dubbed litholapaxy, which along with shock disintegration of bladder stones is the preferred treatment for small calculi today.

The Problems of Urine Retention

Despite a growing body of theoretical knowledge, until the initiation of effective methods of renal replacement little more than a generation ago, people who developed severe kidney problems continued to die. For, after all, failing kidneys are incompatible with long-term survival. Fluid and wastes accumulate in the body. Edema — swelling of the body's tissues — occurs and the patient becomes pale, weak, anemic and breathless. If urine production ceases altogether, he or she develops uremia — a build-up in the body of toxic wastes — and without treatment would die within weeks or even days.

Renal insufficiency may of course be temporary or permanent. A sudden drop in blood pressure due to heart failure or a serious hemorrhage, for instance, may reduce pressure within the glomeruli and compromise the efficiency of filtration. Alternatively, temporary (reversible) kidney damage may result from infection, from illness elsewhere in the body, from drug toxicity or from some blockage in the urinary system which causes obstruction to one or both kidneys.

A common cause of urinary retention in men in later life is prostatic hypertrophy, a condition that occurs when the lobes of the prostate gland, at the base of the bladder, become enlarged and begin to block the flow of urine through the urethra. At first, the flow is slightly reduced; then the patient has to strain to empty his bladder and experiences a "slow stream" with hesitancy in starting urine flow. As the urethra is further compressed, the muscles of the bladder wall thicken and become stronger; the bladder fails to empty completely, and eventually pressure forces urine back up the ureters, so damaging the upper urinary tract and kidneys. As early as 1761, Giovanni Battista Morgagni, an Italian anatomist, discovered the nature of the blockage: through autopsies he found that bladder muscles could so increase in bulk that they look like bundles of cardiac muscle.

Permanent relief did not become available until the 1880s, through surgical removal of the prostate. Before then, the only recourse was to the catheter. These instruments — long tubes that could be gently inserted up the urethra — were certainly known to the Romans, but regained widespread use only at the end of the Middle Ages. Popular materials were gold and silver, which were relatively flexible and provoked less of a reaction, lead and horn (the last was preferred by the Italian surgeon Fabricius of Aquapendente in the sixteenth century). By the end of the seventeenth century, gold had become the material of choice. Experiments with rubber in 1735 proved less than satisfactory; the new substance was sticky in summer and brittle in winter. Further advances came with the flexible metal model with overlap-

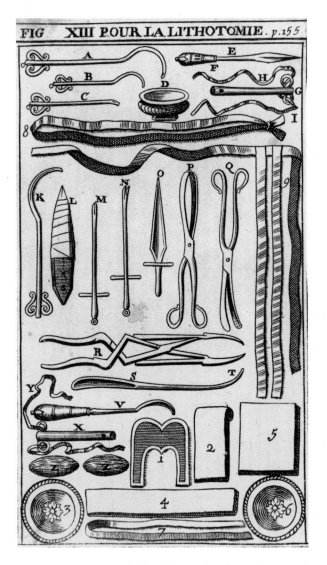

FIG XIII POUR LA LITHOTOMIE. p.155

Requiring the use of a rather gruesome set of instruments, the lithotomy operation was performed usually without an anesthetic for the patient or proper antiseptic precautions.

the surgeon had to make an incision through the perineum into the bladder to insert a catheter.

Ever since it had been observed that eunuchs—males emasculated either through natural deformity or by castration—never developed prostatic hypertrophy, some physicians had suggested that removal of the testes — orchiectomy — might reduce the swollen tissue mass. However, neither this radical solution nor vasectomy achieved the desired end.

Even when such innovative surgeons as George Guthrie and Auguste Mercier inadvertently found the solution in the 1830s by cutting through the obstructing tissue at the neck of the bladder, they saw their procedure only in terms of facilitating catheterization. Removal of the prostate (prostatectomy, developed simultaneously in the United States and Europe) began to gain wide acceptance at the end of the nineteenth century. A simpler solution came in 1912, when the Johns Hopkins surgeon Hugh Young invented his famous "punch operation" to remove only the prostatic tissue pressing on the urethra. Two metal tubes, one inserted inside the other, were introduced into the urethra, and the inner, cutting tube was used to "punch" a hole in the overgrowing tissue, which could then be withdrawn. Today the obstructive tissue can be cut away following direct observation using an endoscope.

Dialysis for Diseased Kidneys

Today the kind of temporary renal episode that would have been fatal before the invention of the artificial kidney can usually be overcome. The patient is kept going on dialysis until his or her own kidneys resume their function. In fact, the original use of the early makeshift kidney machines of the postwar era was merely to support patients in acute, that is temporary, renal failure.

Even at that time the notion of hemodialysis — artificial "cleansing" of the blood — was by no means new. As early as in 1861 an innovative Scot named Thomas Graham described a process he called simply dialysis, showing how crystalloid material was able to diffuse across a semipermeable membrane floating in water. Already dimly perceived was the objective of containing blood in some sort of semipermeable membrane, suspended

ping sections, and, finally, with the vulcanized rubber catheter.

For much of the nineteenth century, then, catheterization became a way of life for many elderly men — although repeated insertion brought with it the risk of kidney infection. For the gentry catheters came in cased sets of seven — one for each day of the week — or they were made to fit into compartments carved in the handles of walking sticks and umbrellas. A Paris goldsmith devised a catheter of silk and gum which could remain *in situ* for up to 10 days.

If the obstruction eventually became too severe for self-catheterization, the lithotomist would be called in. Often by this point, the additional complication of urethral stricture (the narrowing of the passage through scarring) would require the application of a caustic—usually a dilute solution of silver nitrate, although even caustic potash (potassium hydroxide) was tried. If all else failed,

The microdose medical X-ray system requires only a small quantity of radiation to produce a sharp image of bodily organs. Such X rays are now one of the most commonly employed methods of kidney investigation.

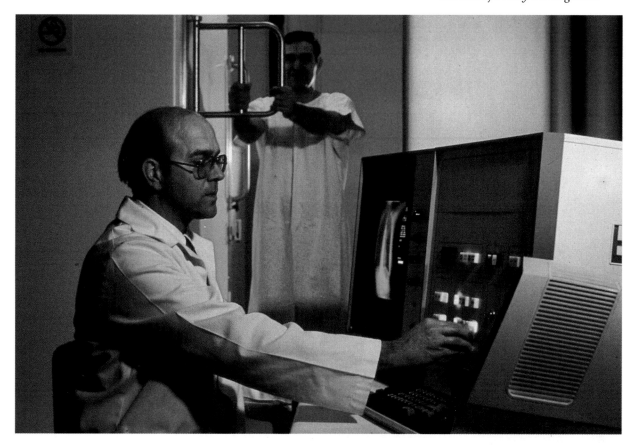

in a fluid medium (now known as dialysate), so that salts and wastes could pass out into the surrounding fluid.

But it was not until 1913 that John J. Abel and his colleagues at Johns Hopkins University made public their work on animals subjected to what was at that time called "vividiffusion" using a prototype artificial kidney. German surgeons performed the first series on humans in 1926. Their greatest problem was to prevent clotting: heparin — an anticoagulant now routinely used during dialysis — had not then been refined.

At the end of World War II it became apparent that several pioneers, working independently, had produced versions of kidney machines. Best-known and most workable of these was the crude apparatus — originally a cellophane tube coiled round a beer can — devised in the Netherlands by Willem Kolff, which became the forerunner of most later machines. Once heparin was freely available

to prevent blood clotting during dialysis, it could be used — for ten to twelve hours at a time two or three times a week — to tide over patients with reversible kidney conditions.

These same patients could alternatively be kept going on peritoneal dialysis. Interest in the use of the peritoneum — the lining of the abdominal cavity — as a dialysing membrane had been mounting over these same decades, and peritoneal dialysis was first performed in 1923. By the 1950s it too had become a viable method of support for patients in acute renal failure.

A few more years were yet to pass, however, before the breakthrough that enabled physicians to save the lives of patients with chronic kidney problems. Overwhelmingly these are people suffering from congenital deformity or from some condition involving progressive loss of kidney tissue. Most common of these are: glomerulonephritis, now believed to be a disorder mediated by the

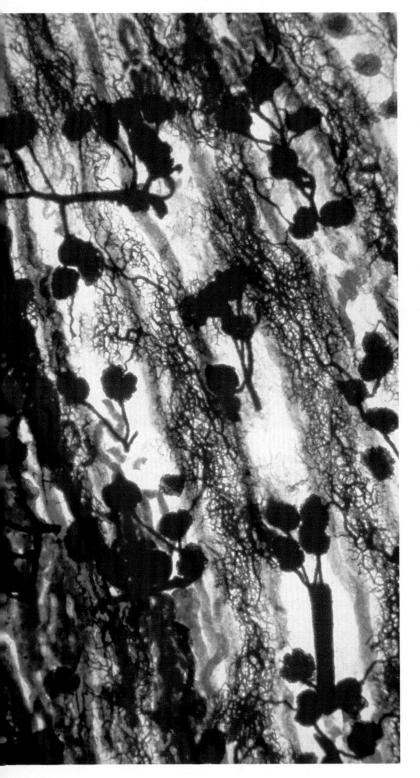

A photomicrograph of the cortex of the kidney reveals the berrylike structures of the glomeruli. The glomeruli filtrate is gradually modified into urine by the tubules which drain into the medulla.

immune system, in which the glomeruli of the nephrons are destroyed; pyelonephritis, a bacterial infection of the kidneys which may become chronic; and polycystic disease, a condition of maldevelopment in which cysts overwhelm the kidney substance. The symptoms of these diseases can be relieved by an unpalatable, low-protein diet, but inevitably the patient's condition worsens. He or she ultimately suffers what is known today as end-stage renal failure (ESRF).

Prior to this, the limiting factor on long-term renal substitution was the problem of access to the blood supply. Blood vessels that are continually punctured with needles begin to break down, until eventually it becomes a major difficulty to find a vein that is both accessible and still resilient enough to support the introduction of a cannula for blood to be tapped off for circulation through the kidney machine. (And indeed there is the same problem with the return of blood to the body through a second cannula.)

The first practicable answer to this came in 1960 with the development of a shunt: two parallel plastic tubes which could be inserted surgically in selected blood vessels in an arm or leg and closed off with a U-connection when not in use. An even more elegant device for securing permanent access was the creation — again in the United States, in 1966 — of an artificial internal connection, or fistula, between the required artery and vein. The shunt, meanwhile, was already enabling physicians to save many patients from a lingering death, and in 1964 specialists in Boston and London began pioneering home dialysis.

Kidney Transplantation

It has of course always been recognized that dialysis is not the ultimate answer to ESRF. Already in the earliest years of this century, the French-American surgeon Alexis Carrel was paving the way for kidney transplants. At the Rockefeller Institute, in addition to conducting experimental kidney transplants in animals (first reported in 1902), Carrel developed the techniques of surgical anastomosis — reconnecting severed blood vessels to reinstate circulation — that are still in use by renal and other surgeons today. But, as Carrel and many of his contemporaries realized, the

Alexis Carrel

Pioneer of Transplantation

The pioneering work which was to gain Alexis Carrel the Nobel Prize in 1912 is said to have been inspired by the murder of French President Carnot, who died when an assassin's bullet severed a main artery.

Vascular surgery was at that time still in its infancy, and such wounds were almost inevitably fatal. Thirty years later, in 1944—the year of his death, aged seventy-one—Carrel's contribution to the field had greatly improved the chances of success in all operations involving vascular repair or surgery.

His education began at a Jesuit school in France, at which he showed an early interest in anatomy by dissecting small birds. It thus came as no surprise to his family when he enrolled to study medicine at the University of Lyon, receiving his degree in 1900.

Inexplicably, he seems then to have lost interest in his studies and emigrated to Canada in 1904 to try his hand at cattle ranching. The venture lasted only briefly, however; medicine once again claimed his attention. It was at the Rockefeller Institute for Medical Research in New York that his interest in the replacement of organs led him to develop a technique for

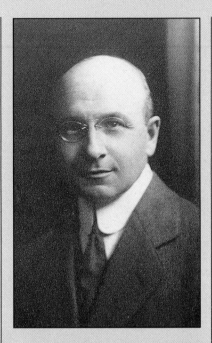

suturing (sewing) blood vessels together end to end with very fine needles to ensure that replaced organs received a constant and adequate blood supply at their new location.

By character rather acerbic and unconventional, Carrel caught popular imagination when, as an extension of his earlier work, he publicly undertook to keep a piece of chicken embryo alive and growing indefinitely.

And indeed, present-day methods in the production of vaccines owe much to his research. Similarly, his joint project with the famous aviator Charles Lindbergh to design a

perfusion pump—a so-called "artificial heart"—to assist in the cultivation of whole organs (a scheme which seemed overly ambitious to many of his peers) led to the construction of apparatus now used in major heart surgery.

He gave distinguished service in the French army during World War I, in particular by devising—with Henry Dakin— an antiseptic which helped to reduce deaths from infected wounds.

His experience of World War II, however, was much less happy; the conclusion of hostilities saw him branded as a traitor. Out of sympathy with Western notions of democracy, he worked for the German-controlled Vichy Government, setting up the Carrel Foundation for the Study of Human Problems. The aims of the institute were very much those that Carrel had previously outlined in his book *Man The Unknown*, published in 1935: that a ruling intellectual elite should use science to benefit the community and confer longevity and spiritual advancement. These were ideals that smacked too strongly of Aryan eugenics and the authoritarianism that the war had been fought to eliminate and, after the French liberation, he was charged with collaboration.

By flushing donor kidneys with fluids, they can be preserved for up to 24 hours before transplantation. This allows time for the selection and transportation of the kidneys to suitable recipients.

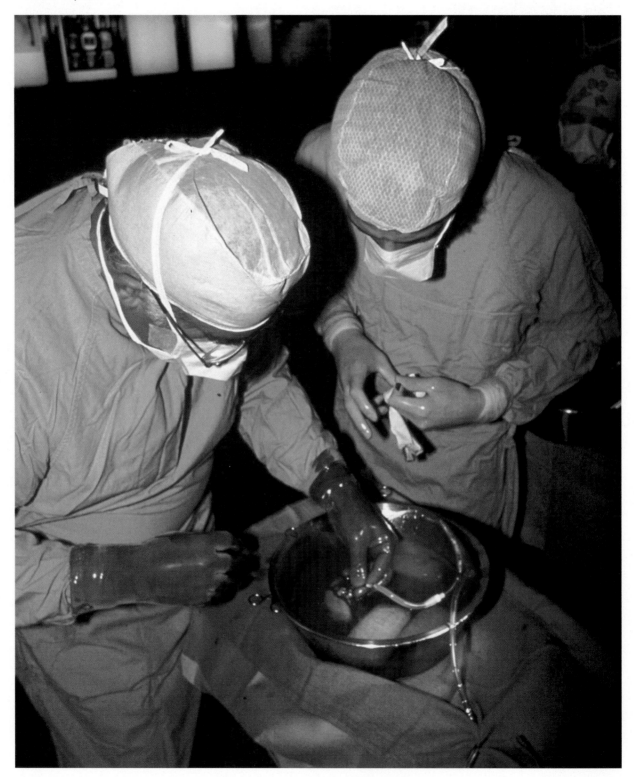

problems associated with tissue rejection were not to be solved so easily.

In fact, a further half century was to elapse before human kidney transplants were pioneered. Following a few isolated attempts at using kidneys from corpses to support dying patients, the first human transplant involving an organ from a live donor — the transfer of a kidney from mother to son — was carried out in France in 1953. Unhappily, tissue rejection set in after the grafted kidney had functioned well for three weeks, and the young man died. A year later surgeons in Boston, Massachusetts, managed to avoid the rejection problem altogether by grafting a kidney from their patient's live identical twin (still the optimum circumstance for organ transplantation). This was the first successful transplant using a live donor.

However, it was not until the introduction of the first generation of immunosuppressive drugs — of which azothiaprine, developed in 1960, was the safest — together with steroids to counteract the graft swelling that accompanies rejection, that kidney transplantation moved out of the realm of epic medicine. Today, with more varied and judicious use of anti-rejection drugs, it is the treatment of choice for most of the forty-per-million new patients per year in Western society who need treatment for end-stage renal failure.

A Disease of the Rich

Gout is an ancient affliction, lamented throughout recorded history. But it was not until 1683 that an English physician, Thomas Sydenham — who suffered its excruciating pain himself — made the clinical distinction between this and other joint disorders in his famous *Treatise on the Gout*. Here, it seemed, was a fashionable disease, affecting the rich or famous — from Charlemagne to Queen Anne, Martin Luther to Lord Nelson.

Although gout may since have lost its glamor, it still retains its characteristic fiery pain and inflammation — both due to a build-up of salt (sodium urate) crystals in the joints; deposits may also occur elsewhere in the body, including in the kidneys (as a kidney stone). Most attacks begin in the big toe, but other joints may be involved, eventually becoming stiff and misshapen.

The exact cause of gout is not known precisely,

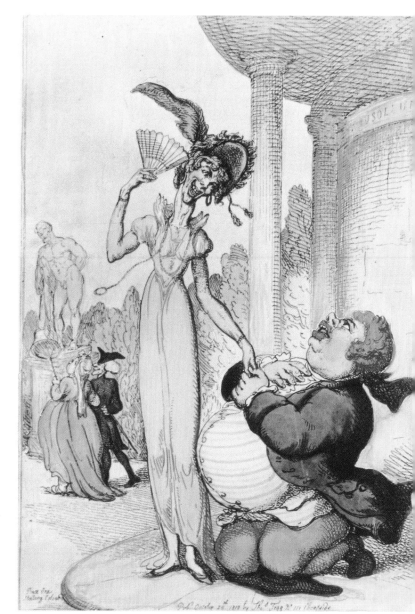

The grossly overweight subject of this political cartoon Dropsy courting Consumption, *by the English caricaturist Thomas Rowlandson, has edema. This abnormal swelling is an important symptom of some kidney diseases, especially those affecting the glomerular filters. Usually the first sign is puffiness around the eyes in the morning, reappearing as puffy ankles by nightfall. If severe, the face and ankles remain swollen and the abdomen becomes distended.*

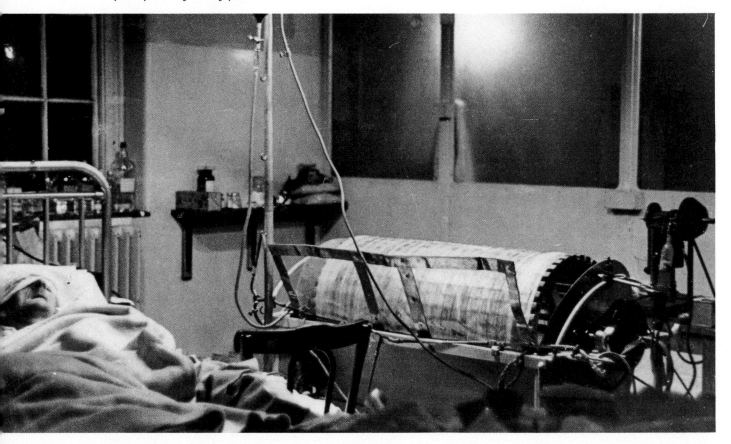

but there is thought to be a hereditary factor at work because this crippling condition often runs in families.

But the real concern is that the disease is an indirect killer. Little more than two decades ago the damage it caused to the kidneys was claiming at least ten thousand lives a year in the United States alone. At this time anti-inflammatory drugs had replaced colchicine (an extract of colchicum, first obtained in 1814) in the treatment of gout. The symptoms were being controlled, but not the consequences.

It was an American research biochemist, Dr George Hutchings, who pioneered the breakthrough that was to save lives. Already Hutchings had three major drug finds to his credit: Daraprim to prevent, or cure, malaria; 6-mercaptopurine (6-MP) to treat leukemia; and the immunosuppressant drug azothiaprine, for use following kidney transplantation operations.

Allopurinol to treat gout evolved as a spin-off from the anti-leukemia drug 6-MP. Allopurinol is a purine compound — previously tried and discarded as a treatment for cancer — which blocks the activity of the substance involved in the metabolic breakdown of the leukemia drug; this same substance (the enzyme xanthine oxydase) converts purines, which are fundamental components of nucleic acids, into the uric acid implicated in the formation of kidney stones. In a classic feat of deduction, Hutchings reasoned that if he could block the enzyme, the level of uric acid in the bloodstream would be greatly reduced.

Clinical trials with allopurinol began at the Duke University Medical Center in Durham, North Carolina, where doctors reported prompt improvement. The results of these trials, published in late 1963, confirmed that kidney stone formation ceased in almost all patients undergoing treatment. From then on, gout has been a curable disorder.

Most modern artificial kidney aids are designed to allow dialysis to take place in the patient's home, permitting them much more flexibility in their way of life. A slow flow of blood trickling through the machine for a six- to eight-hour period, repeated two or three times a week, is enough to keep waste products in the body within safe limits. Because of the time-consuming nature of dialysis, many patients connect themselves to the machine in the late evening, sleep through the night while their blood is being continuously dialyzed, and disconnect themselves in the morning.

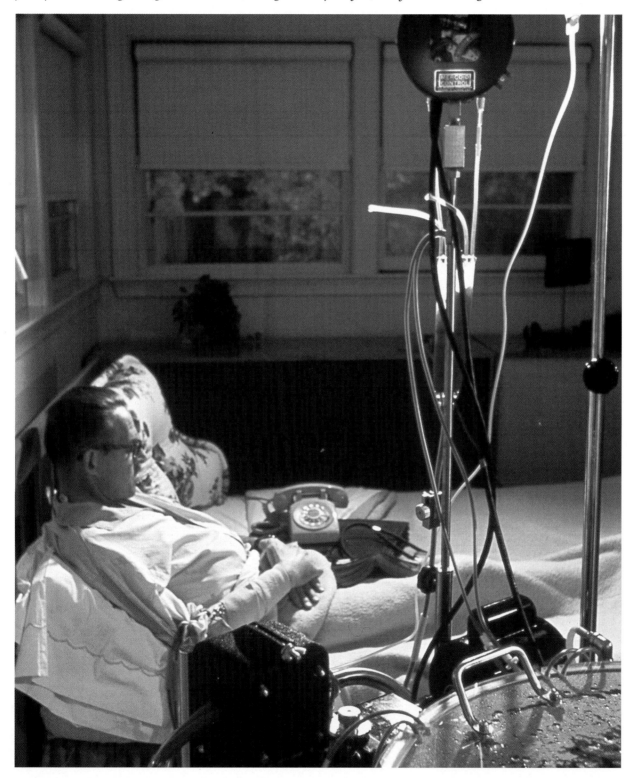

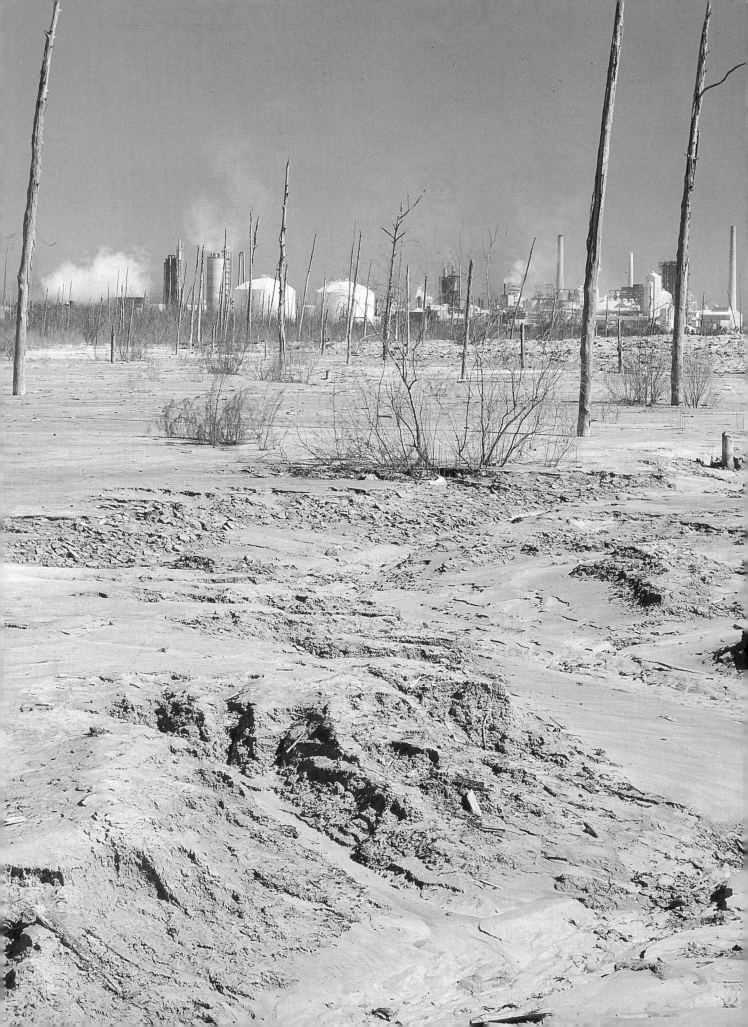

Chapter 2

Fantastic Filters

After eating and drinking, the human body has two principal ways of losing those ingested constituents that are unusable; each is completely different from the other. The first method is the discarding of food residue as feces, the second is the removal of broken down protein and other material in the urine.

As the food we eat is digested and passes through the alimentary tract (the gut), the body absorbs the nutrients that it needs to live and work efficiently. Indigestible fiber (roughage) is left. The body also gets rid of certain substances by putting them back into the roughage, but the bulk of the feces is the food that the body has chosen not to absorb, along with millions of normal bowel bacteria, termed the intestinal flora.

Kidney excretion is completely different. The kidneys do not absorb substances in the way the bowel does. Instead, they filter the by-products of metabolism out of the blood. The gut is thus selective about what it takes in, whereas the kidneys are selective about what they take out.

But why does the body need to excrete at all? Men and women are masters of their own destiny, they can choose what they eat, and the bowel can "choose" what it wants to absorb.

The human body is not a static organ: cells die and need replacing. The substances that make up these cells — and hence the body — are built up mainly from the elements nitrogen, carbon, hydrogen, and oxygen. So also are the by-products left in the body when proteins are broken down.

Carbon and oxygen can be lost as carbon dioxide in the breath during exhalation, and the body can make water from metabolic residues containing hydrogen and oxygen. Both carbon dioxide and water are comparatively easy for the body to expel. But a problem arises when nitrogen has to be excreted. Although in its elemental state it is an inert gas (the air we breathe is eighty per cent nitrogen), the concentrated chemicals produced by the body and known as nitrogenous waste are toxic.

The lifeless landscape around this factory complex in Louisiana sends out a clear signal — the waste products of any chemical system must be removed and disposed of safely, or the system and its surroundings will be poisoned. The human body is superbly equipped with a waste disposal system, but its sophistication goes beyond mere excretion. Built into it is an efficient recycling mechanism, which complements the body's metabolic and other processes.

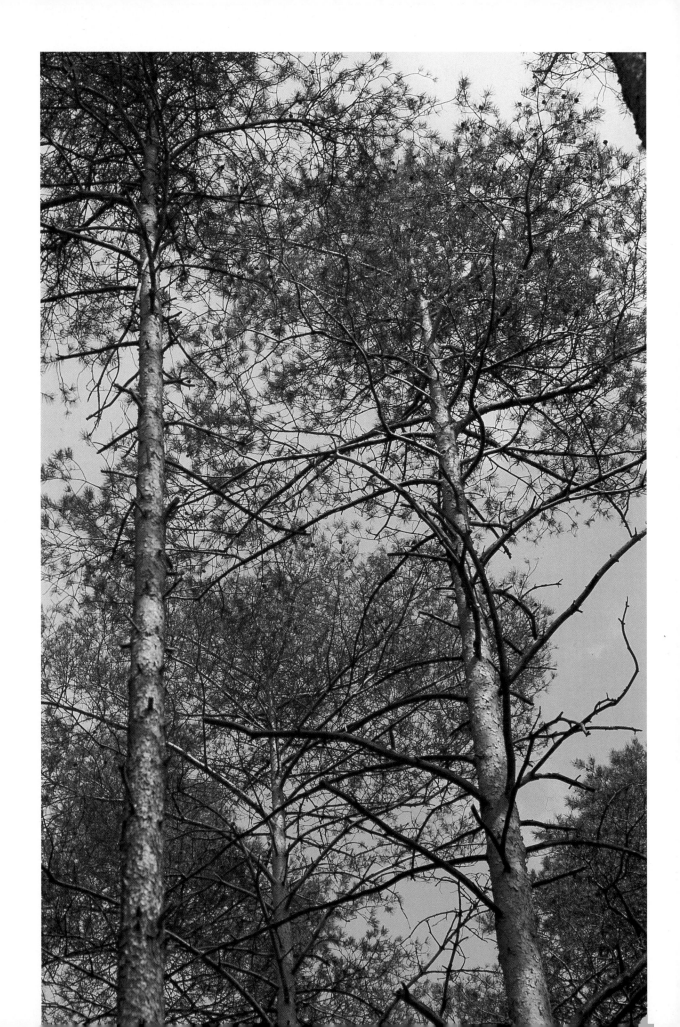

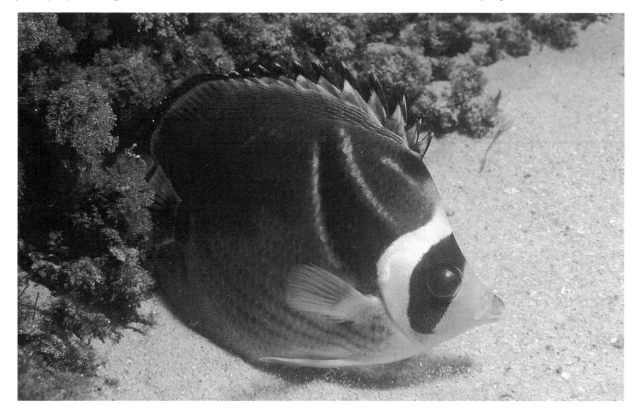

All creatures face the problem of nitrogen excretion, and each species solves it in its own way. Fish excrete nitrogen as ammonia, a poisonous chemical that cannot be stored within the body. But fish have no need to store this waste product, because they can seep out ammonia all the time into their watery environment, where it is rapidly diluted. This method would obviously be completely impractical for a terrestrial and relatively immobile creature.

Birds expel nitrogenous waste as a paste of uric acid (which makes up the white part of the familiar bird dropping). They cannot expel nitrogenous waste as the less toxic substance urea, because this needs to be in very dilute solution and excreted in urine, and flying would be extremely difficult if body weight constantly changed as a bladder filled and emptied.

Earthbound animals, however, are able to store nitrogenous waste in its least toxic form, as urea. This is extracted from the bloodstream by the kidneys and diluted in liquid secretions, to be stored in the bladder as urine. From there it can be intermittently voided.

In addition to ridding the body of certain substances, the kidneys have another role. They also regulate the levels of other normal constituents in the body, particularly of salts and water. Normal daily activities make different demands on the body. For instance, a highly energetic life style results in a high level of metabolic waste in the system; a person may overload the system with salty foods on one day but not on another; the body may need extra water in hot weather to make up for that lost in sweat or through the skin and lungs. And even though the intake of food is fairly selective most of the time, the overall internal balance of all of these substances needs constant adjustment.

The allocation of fluid and metabolites is dictated by the water content of the tissues. A healthy adult may, in the course of one day, take in just over five pints of fluid in food and drink; about half this amount is then lost in urine, about a pint in water

33

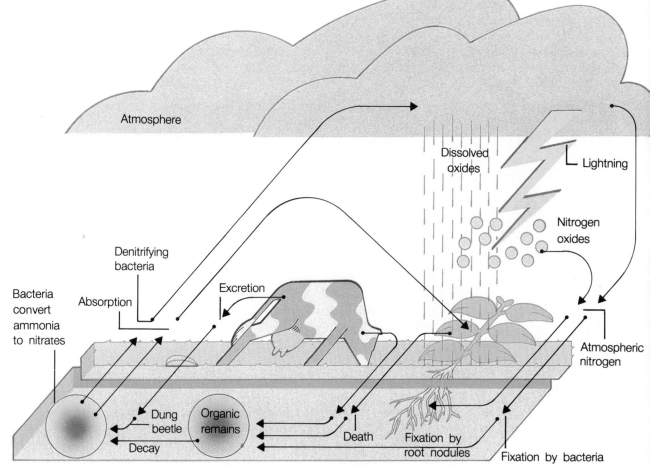

Atmosphere

Dissolved oxides

Lightning

Nitrogen oxides

Denitrifying bacteria

Absorption

Excretion

Bacteria convert ammonia to nitrates

Atmospheric nitrogen

Dung beetle

Organic remains

Decay

Death

Fixation by root nodules

Fixation by bacteria

The nitrogen cycle illustrates well the interdependence of plants, animals and microbes with their environment. Of all life forms, only bacteria and blue-green algae can make use of atmospheric nitrogen, converting it into a form that is usable by plants. The roots of certain plants, such as legumes, can also utilize atmospheric nitrogen, because they contain nitrogen-fixing bacteria. Lightning, too, fixes atmospheric nitrogen, which enters the soil dissolved in rain water. From the soil, nitrogen provides nourishment for plants, which return it to the soil after they die or are eaten. There the nitrogen passes to lower creatures, such as the dung beetle, and other bacteria which release it back into the atmosphere to maintain the cycle.

vapor from the lungs, another pint in perspiration, and the rest by way of the gut. But when the body temperature has been raised, more fluid is lost through the skin and lungs. Unless that fluid is replaced immediately by drinking large amounts of water, the blood becomes concentrated and the tissues become dehydrated.

A Collecting System

The urinary tract is composed of the two kidneys, a ureter connected to each one, the bladder, and the urethra which leads to the outside world.

The kidneys are paired organs; both work separately but their functions are the same. We have two kidneys — much as we have two lungs and two legs — because we are largely symmetrical creatures. One kidney is not there just in case the other ceases to function, although some people do have only one kidney and yet lead a normal life because it functions adequately alone.

The kidneys lie at the back of the abdominal wall on each side of the backbone (spinal column) and are highly vascular organs, with many blood vessels. They are well protected by the ribs, under

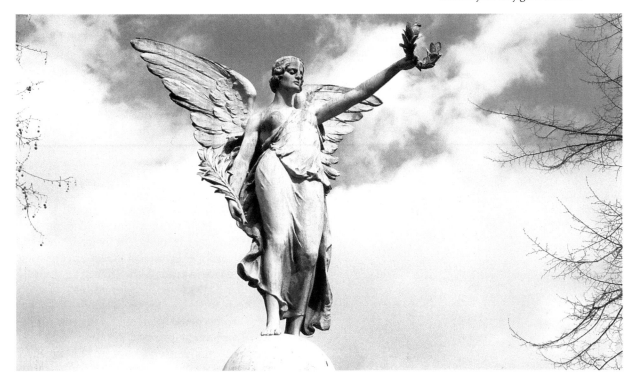

which they nestle, and by the muscles of the abdomen and back. Each kidney is surrounded by a thick capsule of fat which further protects it, also insulating it against excessive heat loss.

The kidneys are located thus at the center of the body, because they need to be connected to two of the most important blood vessels: the main vessel leading away from the heart (the aorta) and the one back to it (the inferior vena cava). They process well over two thousand pints of blood every day, and have to be right next to these main thoroughfares of blood. The renal arteries, usually one for each kidney, come directly off the aorta. Each plunges into the center of the kidney (the hilus). Beside it the renal vein emerges to join the inferior vena cava. Because blood enters the kidneys so near to the heart, without any length of narrowing vessels to reduce the rate of flow, the kidneys have to be able to withstand tremendous pressure. For this reason, the tough fibrous coat that surrounds each organ remains tense.

Each kidney is on average about four and a half inches long. A man's kidney weighs about five ounces and a woman's about half an ounce less.

The top of each kidney is larger than the base, and each tips forward at the top toward the main blood vessels. The left kidney is flanked by the pancreas, the jejunum and part of the colon. The right kidney touches against the duodenum and colon, and is located lower than the left one because the large mass of the liver displaces it downward. Both kidneys move up and down when a person breathes, and both move nearly an inch lower when a person stands. In most people it is not possible to feel the kidneys through the abdominal wall, although in a thin person with loose abdominal muscles one can usually be felt.

On top of each kidney sits a suprarenal, or adrenal, gland. These glands are part of the endocrine system, and each has a slightly different shape; the right one looks like a tricorn hat, and the left one looks like a half moon. In both the concavity wraps around the top of the kidney.

From the center of the kidney the ureter emerges as a funnel-shaped tube. The top end lies within the kidney, where it is called the pelvis (having no bearing whatsoever, apart from identical etymology, on the pelvis of the skeleton). To avoid

MAIN ORGANS
OF THE
URINARY SYSTEM

- Kidney
- Ureter
- Bladder

confusion in the following descriptions, this pelvis in the kidney is referred to as the renal pelvis, and the large circle of bone at the base of the spinal column is referred to as the skeletal pelvis.

From the renal pelvis the ureters lead as a tube down the back wall of the abdomen, behind the intestines until they reach the skeletal pelvis. Here they dip down into the circle of bone and run forward and enter the bladder through its muscular wall. (A few people have two ureters coming from one kidney.)

The bladder is an expandable bag made from a basketwork of interlacing involuntary muscle. The muscle fibers run in whorls, and sweep up and down from the apex to the neck of the bladder. This intricate and unique layout of fibers means that when the muscles contract, the hole (the internal meatus) at the base of the bladder opens.

When the bladder is empty, it collapses down behind the front of the skeletal pelvis (the pubic bone, low down at the front of the abdomen), and as it fills it gradually rises above this bone. The movement is often quite noticeable in a child, because in children the bladder lies higher above the pelvis than it does in an adult.

The bladder can usually contain about half a pint of urine before it requires voiding. A healthy bladder can contain nearly a pint, but when it is this full reflex contractions in the detrusor muscle make the urge to urinate difficult to ignore. However, the bladder possesses the ability to stretch to a much greater size, and in conditions that involve chronic outflow obstruction, the bladder can increase its dimensions sufficiently to hold up to three and a half pints or more of fluid.

The inside of the bladder is made up of a membrane folded and wrinkled across the surface, except for one piece of smooth tissue in the form of a triangle. This is called the trigone, with the openings of the ureters at the two upper points and the exit from the bladder to the urethra at the base point.

Although the muscles of the bladder itself are not under voluntary control, the muscles of the pelvic floor are and emptying the bladder can thus also be controlled. There is still some controversy about exactly what voluntary relaxation preempts voiding, but there is strong evidence that it is not caused

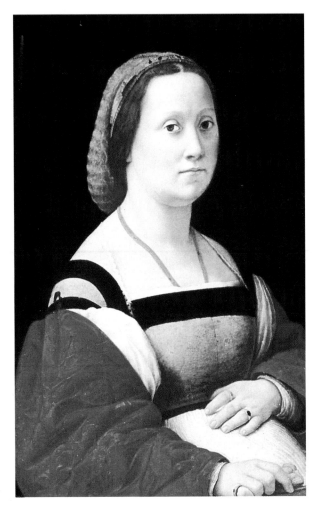

As the bladder fills with urine, it rises above the pubic bone. This movement is restricted during pregnancy, reducing the capacity of the bladder so that frequent urination becomes necessary.

simply by the relaxation of a band of muscle (vesical sphincter) at the neck of the urethra. A few seconds before urination the pelvic floor drops and the vesical sphincter relaxes along with the other muscles. Urine enters the urethra as the detrusor muscles in the wall of the bladder contract involuntarily and expel the urine through the urethra.

Urine is not forced back up the ureters when the bladder contracts — or at any other time — because the angle at which they enter the bladder ensures that contraction automatically closes the orifices off. It is usually possible to override the desire to urinate — even while actually urinating — by voluntarily contracting the pelvic and sphincter muscles, which in turn makes the detrusor muscle relax again.

The bladder fills with urine at different rates according to many external factors. At night far less urine is produced than during the day. But a night-shift worker voids three times a night and once during daylight hours. It takes about a week for the production of urine to readjust once a worker moves onto the day shift. Many people experience similar inconveniences when jet-lagged after traveling across several time zones.

The Exit Route

Urine leaves the bladder through a single tube, the urethra. A woman's urethra is just over an inch and a half long, and its sole purpose is to provide this exit route. It has a ring of muscle, or sphincter, to prevent leakage of urine. A man's urethra is much longer, at seven to eight inches and, unlike a woman's, it has a dual role — both excretory and reproductive.

As the male urethra leaves the bladder it becomes the prostatic urethra, because its walls there comprise the prostate gland. The internal structure of the prostate is part of the reproductive system. It is from this point on that the male urethra has two functions, because the ejaculatory duct joins the urethra within the prostate gland. Sperm is prevented from entering the bladder by the same structure that stops the urine from entering the semen — the sphincter vesicae — which is made up from the sweeps of detrusor muscle in the bladder. Urine is deadly to sperm and some experts

believe that an extra safeguard is provided by the bulbourethral, or Cowper's, glands which open into the urethra an inch or so below the ejaculatory duct. These glands secrete fluid into the semen during ejaculation, and it is thought that this fluid may neutralize the spermicidal property of any urine still lingering in the urethra.

Although the female urethra has no reproductive role, it contains some vestiges from a time before the embryonic male and female organs are differentiated. The urethral glands are sometimes referred to as the "female Prostate," even though the tissue is not similar when studied under the microscope. The wall of the urethra contains erectile layers along with muscular and mucous layers — in fact they have exactly the same structure as the male urethra.

The walls of the female urethra remain in contact, and the end farthest from the bladder is just a small slit when urine is not being passed. For women the use of detergent in bath water, say in the form of a bubble bath, reduces the surface tension of the water. The force holding the ends of the urethra

37

*While the body is active, it produces
more urine than when it is relaxed,
and while asleep the rate of
production is lowest. This pattern
can be disturbed by certain factors,
such as shiftwork.*

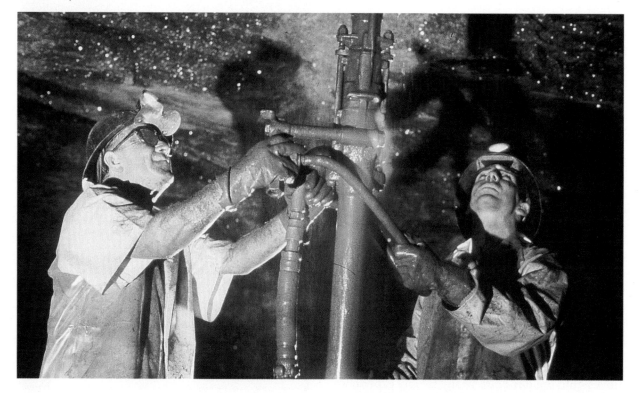

together is lost, allowing a little detergent to enter. This may manifest itself as bubbles in the urine.

As mentioned previously, many experts do not believe in the existence of a thick band of sphincter muscle at the base of the bladder, but instead consider the pelvic floor muscles to have an important role in bladder control. If this is so, it explains why women who have given birth to several children often lose the tone of these pelvic floor muscles, and suffer from "stress" incontinence — the leaking of urine during coughing, laughter or exercise. Upward pressure on the bladder overcomes the pressure holding urine in, and so a spurt of urine passes along the urethra until the pressures equalize. The shortness of the female urethra also accounts for the higher incidence of urinary infections and bladder inflammation such as cystitis among women.

The Miniature Filter Plant

The kidney itself has an intricate structure. It is divided into separate regions, packed into which are more than one million nephrons, functioning structures so minute it is hard to imagine that each acts as a tiny filter.

The outer layer nestling beneath the fibrous coat is called the cortex, and fingers of this push down into the body of the kidney. Between the fingers lies the medulla, which is different in appearance because it contains different parts of the filtering units. Running up from the funnel-shaped end of the ureter to meet the medulla are urine-collecting tubes or calyces, which branch and disperse into the body of the organ. The bulges of medulla between the calyces, the papillae, collect urine from as many as seventy thousand nephrons.

The shape of these calyces is occasionally cast in perfect detail by what is known as a staghorn kidney stone. As the stone grows over the years, it fills the top of the renal pelvis and eventually the calyces, giving it the form of antlers or branched coral. Urine enters the healthy calyces through the ducts of Bellini, which are shaped like minute slits, allowing them to close if pressure builds up in the kidney so that urine cannot flow back.

The purpose of the kidney is to filter the blood,

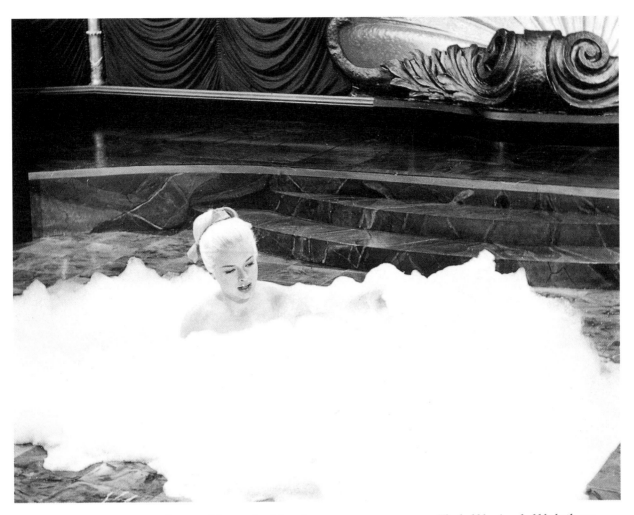

and it is important to understand how the blood enters the kidney before considering the equipment needed for filtering.

The renal artery leaves the aorta and divides into five branches, which fan out on reaching the renal pelvis in order to supply five distinct areas of the kidney. They are known as "end arteries" because they do not join with any other vessel. This factor is important anatomically because should such an artery become blocked, the piece of tissue it serves would not be able to receive blood from any other source and would die. About one person in three has one or all of these branches coming directly off the aorta and entering the segments within the kidney themselves.

Once inside the kidney, the arteries branch again and again as they travel up the pyramids of the medulla, until they reach the edge of the cortex. There the arteries fan out, and smaller branches lead off at right angles to feed every part of the cortex. These tiny interlobular arteries give rise to the even smaller arterioles, which go to form the tangle of capillaries known as the glomerulus. It is

The bubbles in a bubble bath are formed by detergent action, which reduces the surface tension of the water. In the absence of surface tension, the urethra can admit traces of detergent.

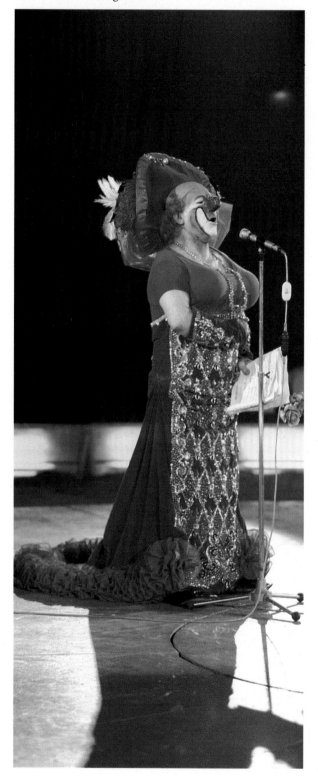

in the glomerulus of the kidney that the actual filtration occurs.

The glomerulus sits inside the top of a tubule made up of separate portions, each with a different function. At the top of each nephron is a cup-shaped structure known as Bowman's capsule. The actual filter is the glomerular basement membrane, which acts as a barrier between the capillaries and the urinary space. It is made of a mat of filaments which, on the Bowman's capsule side, interlock with one another like the teeth of two combs pressed together. Gaps known as "slit pores" between the teeth allow comparatively small molecules to pass through but nothing as large as blood corpuscles can normally cross the membrane into the urinary space. The fluid pressure in the capillaries is much greater than that of the urinary space, and plasma and smaller protein molecules are pushed through because of this irresistible pressure gradient.

The basement membrane offers a large surface area for filtration and an astonishing three fluid ounces of liquid pass through the membrane every minute. Glucose, amino acids, phosphates, sodium and chlorides pass through the filter too. But because the body requires these substances, and much of the fluid that passes into the urinary space, the kidney is able to reabsorb many of the components according to the specific needs of the body at any one time. It works on the same principle as a woman sorting out her purse. She pours all the contents onto a table, puts back the things she needs — such as keys, money and cosmetics — and sweeps any garbage into a bin.

The Bowman's capsule gives way to a winding tube called the proximal tubule. The cells lining it are unlike those in any other area of the nephron because, instead of being flat, interlocking cells, they have brush borders which greatly increases the surface area of the tubule. These numerous microvilli and the presence of many mitochondria (a cell's power plant) indicate that this is an area in which energy-consuming reactions are actively occurring. In fact eighty per cent of the water filtered out of the blood is reabsorbed by this portion of the nephron, along with eighty per cent of the sodium that has passed through the filter.

Encircling the tubule are the thousands of tiny

In its fertile past, this dry river bed
and its surrounding catchment area
in the Navaho Desert would have
functioned like the network of veins
that arise from smaller "tributaries"
within the kidneys.

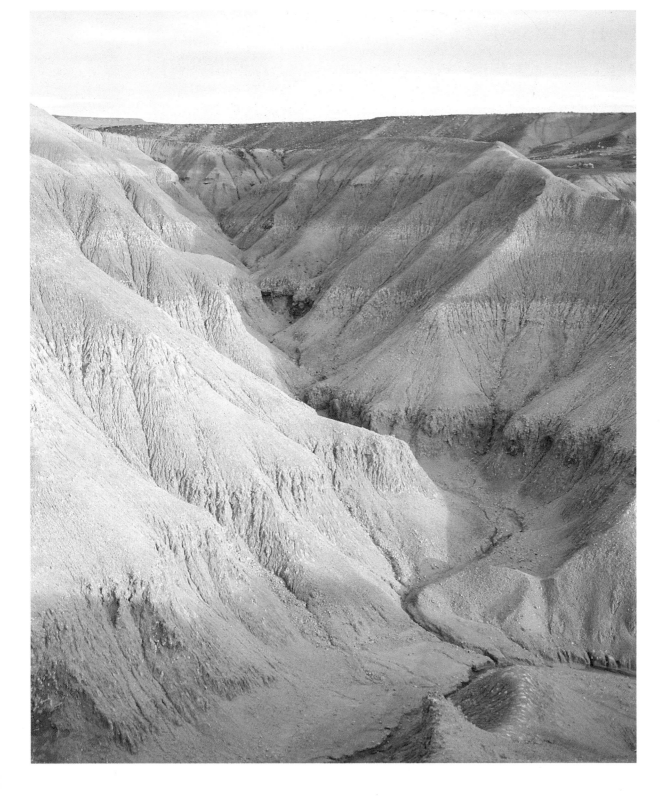

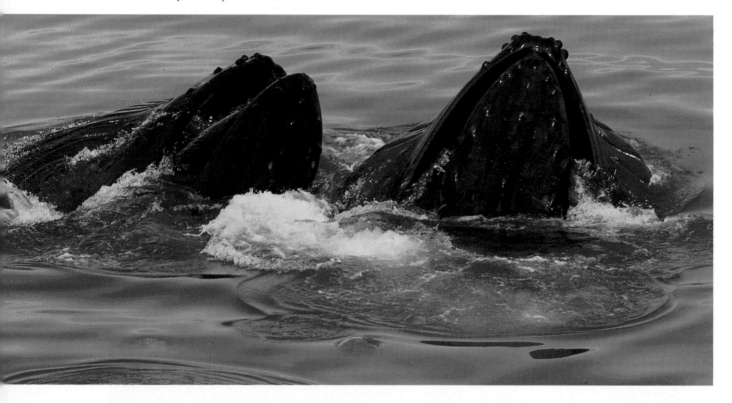

vessels ready to receive the reabsorbed elements and transport them back through the venous system. They are known as stellate veins because of their star shape, and the blood — rejuvenated with water and salts — travels back through an enlarging network of veins to the renal pelvis of the kidney. From there it passes to the renal vein and then joins the inferior vena cava on its journey to the heart, from where it is pumped to the lungs for reoxygenation.

Meanwhile, back at the nephron, the developing urine passes from the proximal convoluted tubule into a downward-sweeping loop, the loop of Henle. This delves down into the medulla of the kidney and rises back into the cortex. Metabolically the descending portion of the loop is functionless, and water passes through the wall by simple osmosis (the passage of water from a weak solution to a strong solution through a membrane until both solutions have the same strength). As urine rises up the other side of the loop, it comes under the influence of actively ion-pumping cells. Here sodium is pumped out back into the blood.

The length of the loop is very variable — in seven out of eight people they are relatively short — about an inch long — and it is only the long loops that dip right down into the papillae of the kidney. The urine in the tube becomes more concentrated as it passes downward because water and salts continue to seep back through the walls of the nephron, which are thin in this area. On the upward part of the loop the cells are thicker, fat cells without a brush border, and it is believed that this part is responsible for the exchange of ions such as sodium and chloride.

The nephron has another portion of convoluted tubule at the other end of the loop of Henle, just before it joins with the collecting tubule. The walls of the collecting tubules gradually taper, increasing in thickness as they reach the papillae of the kidney.

Scientists believe that these collecting tubules show a unique response to antidiuretic hormone (ADH), one of the many chemical messengers secreted by the pituitary gland. Under the influence of this hormone, the cuboidal epithelial cells that

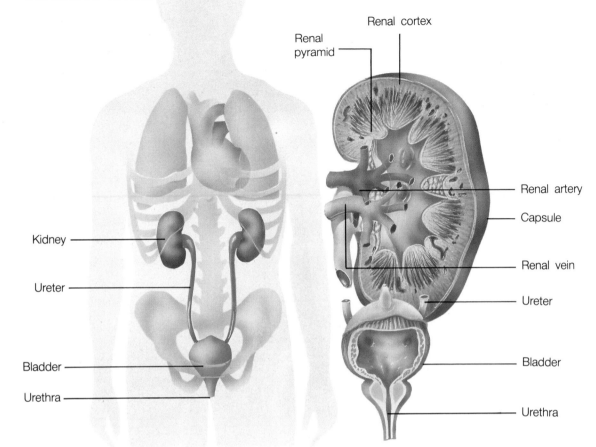

The kidney performs the vital function of separating dissolved waste from the blood, and also maintains the balance of salts, water and trace elements in the body. Its purpose, therefore, is essentially filtration. It has a large supply of blood — via the renal arteries which branch down to capillaries that disperse the blood in the cells of the kidney. The purified blood is returned to the body through the renal veins, and the liquid waste passes to the renal pelvis, down the ureter and into the bladder to be voided.

line the tubules become permeable to water. This allows it to pass from within the tubule to the surrounding papillae, so continuing the concentration process of the urine. If the hormone is not present in the blood, however, the walls become "waterproof" and the urine in the tubules therefore remains dilute.

Just before reaching the top of each papilla, the collecting tubules join together to form the ducts of Bellini. The papillae also contain the lowest portion of the hairpin loop of Henle before the tubule sweeps back up to the cortex again, so this area of the kidney has two separate structures available to reabsorb water and concentrate the urine. It is known as the counter-current mechanism. If the renal papilla is not functioning correctly, the urine leaves the proximal tubule overdiluted and full of sodium. This vulnerable area of the kidney bears the brunt of any infection or damage from chemicals or drugs.

The collecting tubules join up to form the renal papilla, which sits in a calyx in the renal pelvis, and it is from the calyces that the waves of muscular

Hydroponics is a method of growing plants without soil. The nutrients are supplied in water and selectively taken into the roots. In a similar way salts are regulated and urine separated in the kidney.

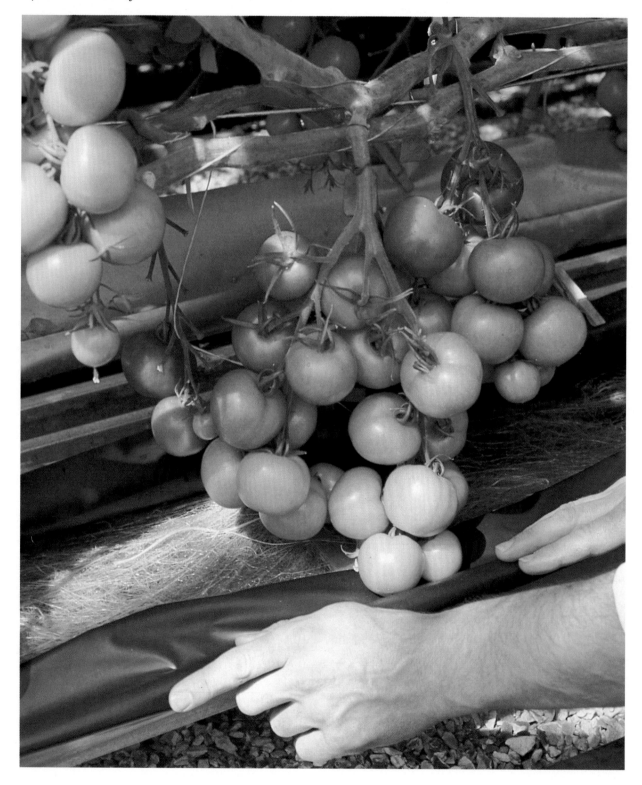

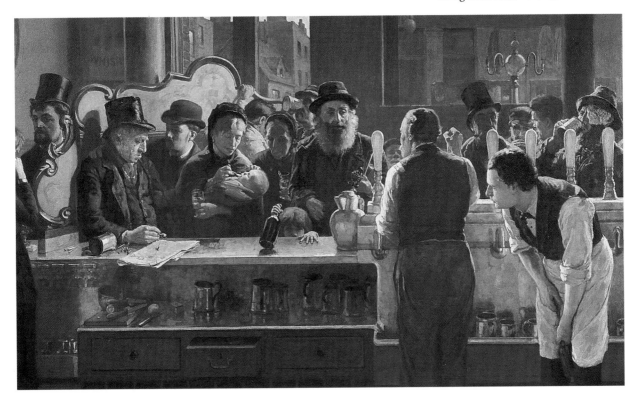

contraction (peristalsis) occur that squeeze the urine out of the kidneys and down the ureters. The muscles of the calyces are involuntary, and scientists believe that the contractions are triggered off by distention in the tubules, which causes each adjacent muscle cell to contract in a manner similar to the way the muscles of the heart work. (Most other muscles of the body are stimulated by a ganglion or nerve cell.) Once the peristaltic waves have been initiated, they travel down the full length of the ureters.

Certain disorders of the kidney can prevent the walls of the calyces from touching because they become congested with urine. This overrides the automatic peristaltic action, but urine still travels to the bladder under the influence of gravity and filtration pressure.

The Biological Freeway

This complicated anatomy of the kidney can best be understood by picturing all the elements present in a drop of blood as it travels along the aorta for distribution around the body. The blood is like a full motorbus heading down the freeway of the aorta. Like any freeway, there are few turnoffs along the route and the motorbus travels fast. It is full; aboard are the wealthy red blood cells rich with oxygen, white blood cells, platelets and plasma proteins such as albumin and transferrin. Other passengers are the alpha, beta and gamma globulins, salts broken down into ions of sodium, chloride, potassium, calcium, bicarbonate, phosphate and many others; molecules of glucose; steroids and hormones; and nitrogenous waste.

The motorbus leaves the freeway and heads off along the renal artery toward the kidney. Once in the kidney, progress slows down because the route is now more like the narrow, twisting streets of a small town. Finally the arterioles narrow still further until they are only one cell thick — these are the capillaries.

The first "stop" is the glomerulus. Here the walls are so thin that the occupants of the motorbus can look through them into the urinary space beyond. Together with the nephron below it acts as a sort of pedestrian area where some of the travelers can get

*A snake propels itself along by waves
of muscular contraction. Another
muscular wave action, called
peristalsis, occurs in the ureters to
squeeze urine along from the kidneys
to its storage place in the bladder.*

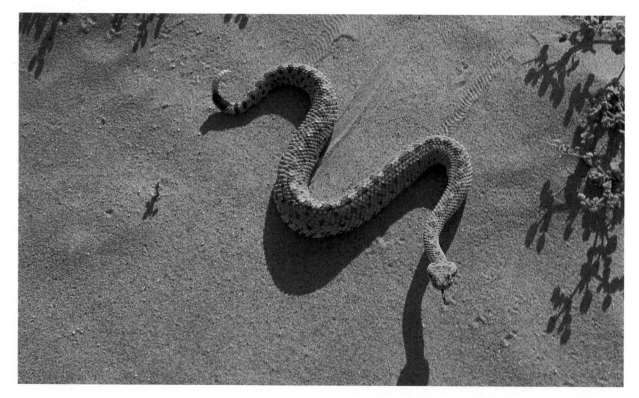

off. The motorbus has to pass on round the area, carrying the passengers who are too large to get off the bus.

Into the area go most of the salt ions, such as sodium and potassium, along with the nitrogenous waste, glucose and a great deal of water. The motorbus carries on around the outside of the nephron, but the rich red blood cells are having to pay for the extra travel by handing out their oxygen. The kidney is involved in active excretion and reabsorption as well as passive filtration, and the tissues of the organ need oxygen and glucose for energy.

The motorbus reaches the capillaries outside the tubule, and here half of the passengers who got off and went into the pedestrian area have the chance to get back on again at a number of different places around the outside of the nephron. Eighty per cent of the sodium ions get left in the area outside the proximal convoluted tubule, but eighty per cent of the filtered water goes back on the motorbus. At the stop outside the loop of Henle both water and sodium leave the area and rejoin the motorbus. At

the stop outside the ascending loop of Henle sodium is exchanged for potassium and hydrogen ions. The last opportunity to take on passengers comes at the collecting tubules which are sometimes "open" and sometimes "shut." If the hormone environment is correct, water can leave the pedestrian area and travel back on the motorbus; but if it is not, the water must stay within the urinary system.

The motorbus then continues on its way back toward the renal vein. It has offloaded all its heavier passengers and is now a group of poorer (deoxygenated) red corpuscles, along with the correct mixture and concentration of ions. The white blood cells and platelets, plasma proteins and immune globulins all came along just for the ride and have not changed at all. The motorbus rejoins the freeway back toward the heart with all the rest of the deoxygenated blood.

But what is happening back at the pedestrian area? The motorbus has carefully left behind all the trouble-makers — the nitrogenous waste in the form of urea, most of the potassium ions and some

46

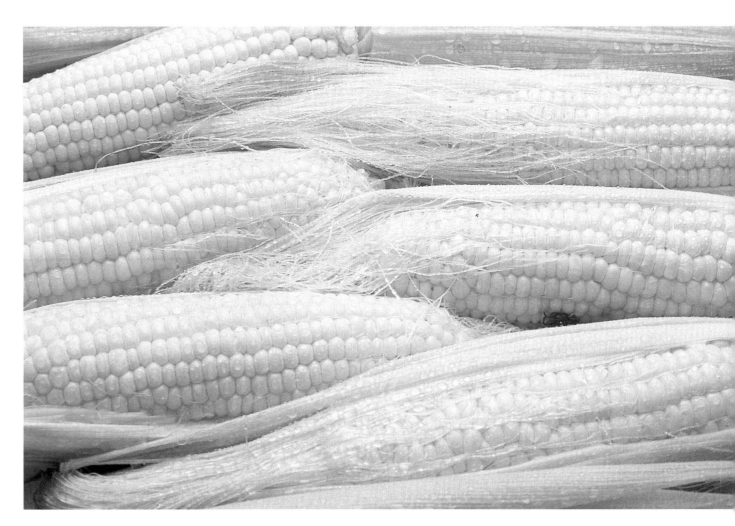

of the sodium ions, and other unnatural substances such as drugs. From here the unwanted components of the blood are washed away down the ureters and into the bladder for eventual expulsion.

Some salts and water are lost through sweat along with traces of urea, but sweating is primarily part of the body's cooling system. The fact that sweat contains some of the same constituents as urine should not lead to the erroneous supposition that sweat glands in any way control or regulate the levels of toxins in the blood.

One curious side aspect of the loss of certain chemicals in sweat is that some ingested substances such as curry can be smelt on the skin (strongly under a watch strap for example) but not in the urine, and that other ingested foods such as asparagus produce a pungent smell in the urine but no scent on the skin.

The nerves that supply the kidney and ureters are out of the orbit of voluntary control by the central nervous system because they are part of the autonomic nervous system. The fibers that wrap around the blood vessels of the kidney and the

The arrangement of nephrons and their collecting tubules in the kidney appears like grains of corn on the cob. This convoluted type of arrangement gives a large surface area, which is important in the kidney for ensuring maximum collecting capacity.

Fanning increases the evaporation of perspiration on the skin and cools the body, ridding it of some of its salts. Unlike the excretory process in the kidney, this loss can have adverse effects, such as causing cramps.

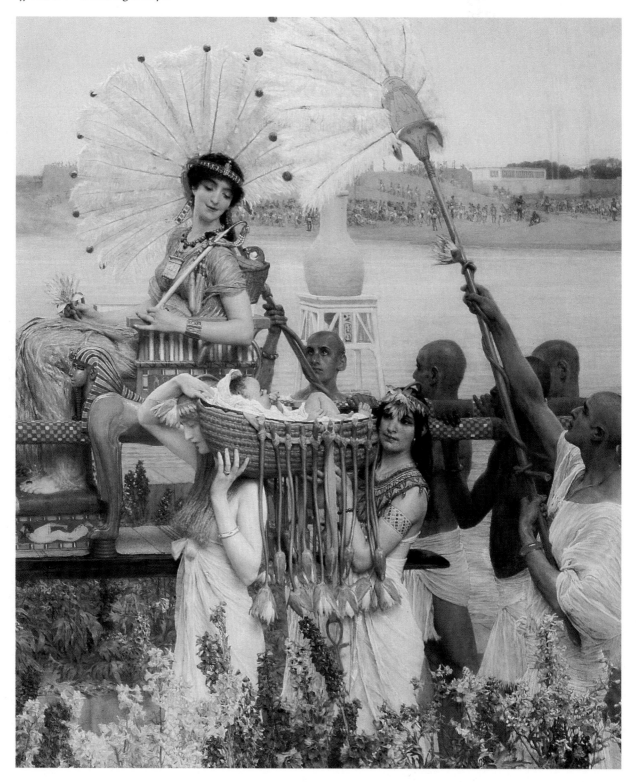

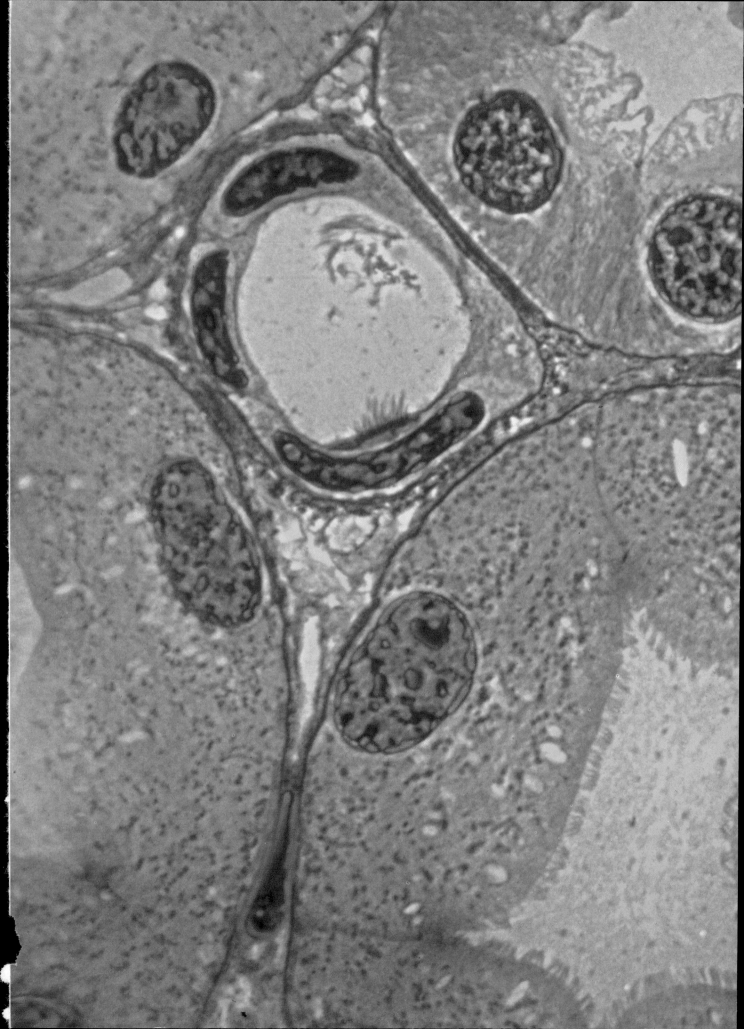

The miraculous intricacy of human body structures is nowhere better demonstrated than in the kidneys. These paired organs are located high up toward the rear of the abdomen, partly protected by the lower ribs.

They are supplied with blood by the renal arteries, which branch off the aorta, the main vessel carrying blood from the heart. Blood cleansed of wastes by the kidneys' filters is returned to the circulation via the

renal veins. The wastes, in solution in urine, pass down the ureters and into the bladder. The nearest neighbors of the kidneys are the adrenal glands, which secrete various hormones.

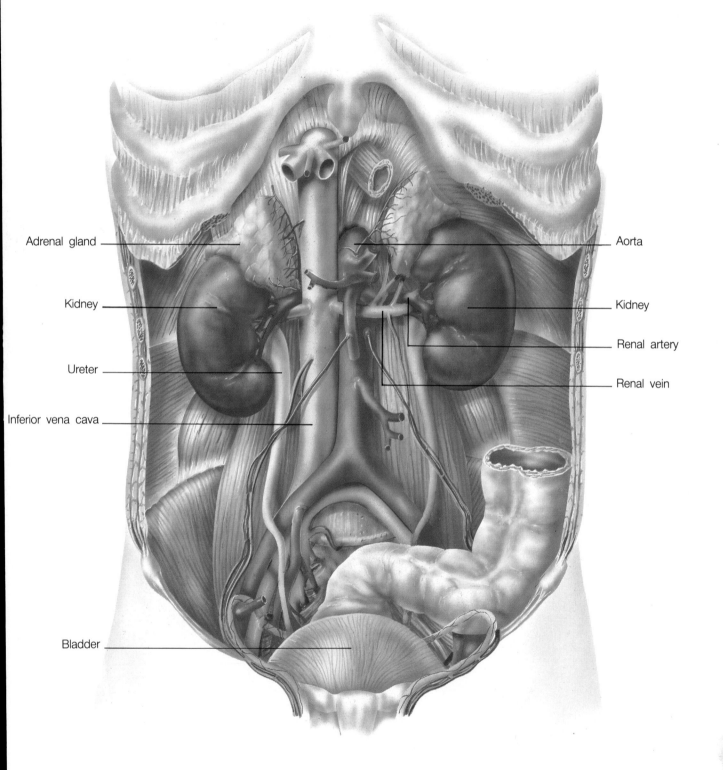

Adrenal gland

Kidney

Ureter

Inferior vena cava

Bladder

Aorta

Kidney

Renal artery

Renal vein

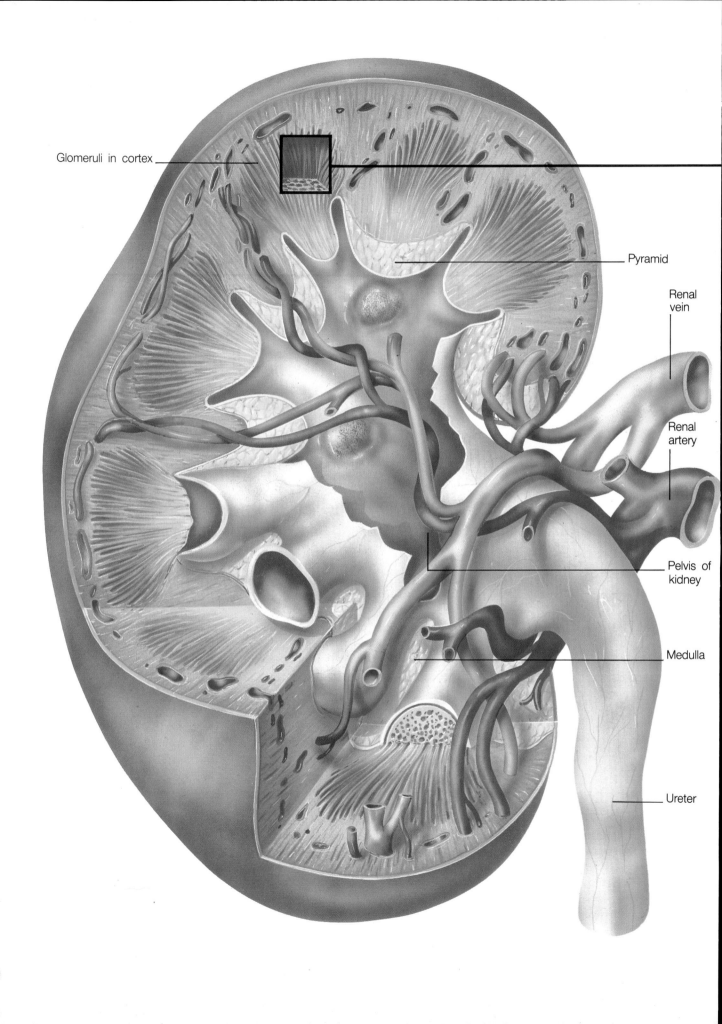

Glomeruli in cortex

Pyramid

Renal vein

Renal artery

Pelvis of kidney

Medulla

Ureter

The kidneys are protected by the spine and lower ribs, but they can be injured by forceful blows. Even more at risk are the ureters, which can be cut by pelvic fractures or by a mishap during surgery.

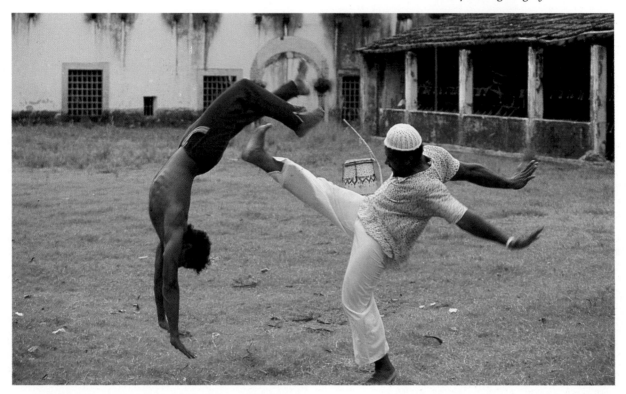

organ itself originate from a mass of interconnecting nerve fibers known as the celiac plexus, the largest of the great autonomic plexuses. Filaments from this plexus run down taking in filaments from other ganglions and nerves until they regroup and interchange to form the renal plexus. The fibers from here run around the renal artery and vein, and then travel on into the body of the kidney to supply the glomeruli and tubules — particularly those within the cortex of the kidney.

Most of the renal nerves are concerned with motor impulses, not sensory ones. The human kidneys work, but no sensation can be felt coming directly back from them. Peristaltic waves cannot be felt passing along the ureters, for example, and should a calculus, or stone, become lodged in the ureter the pattern of pain sensation is not specific, as it is if a piece of bone gets stuck in the throat. The renal plexus also supplies fibers to the ureters and testicles or ovaries.

Sympathetic nerve fibers also supply the bladder. Parasympathetic nerves come from the pelvic splanchnic nerves, and take motor impulses to the muscular wall. They also carry inhibitory impulses to the vesical sphincter muscle. There are sensory fibers in the bladder, and messages travel back to the brain giving information on the fullness of the bladder which impinges on consciousness.

A System at Risk?

Each kidney is protected not only by the ribs but also, in adults, by the coat of perirenal fat that surrounds it. In peacetime open injuries to the kidney are a rare occurrence; those that do happen usually result from stabbings or shootings. The kidney is also vulnerable to injury if a person is involved in a traffic accident. Ribs fractured during crushing injuries can lacerate the tough outer capsule of the kidney, but the organ has an incredible healing ability because of the generous blood supply it receives. Often a split in the kidney, through the cortex and right down into the calyx, heals with little or no loss of kidney function. Occasionally tiny clots of blood remain within the organ after an injury. The blood supply to part of the kidney is impaired, so the organ does not

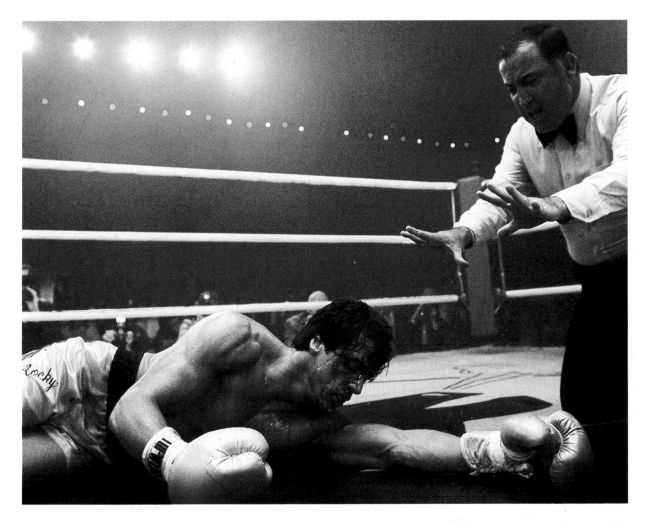

receive enough oxygen and becomes ischemic, leading eventually to high blood pressure (hypertension).

The ureters are at risk during pelvic surgery, when they can be accidentally cut. Sometimes the bladder is cut and urine collects in the abdomen or (in women) leaks from the vagina. In both cases the usual treatment is to repair the damage just as soon as possible.

The bladder may also be injured by trauma to the pelvis; it may rupture if full at the moment of injury or be lacerated by particles of bone from an injury. The urethra itself is also at risk during any injury to the pelvis of the skeleton, and treatment varies from immediate surgery to a more conservative management, draining the bladder and leaving the urethra alone for six weeks. Unfortunately injury to the proximal urethra results in impotence in thirty per cent of men, and in others recovery can take up to two years.

Another classic injury to a different portion of the male urethra is caused by falling astride a bar or a post. This used to be a common injury in the days of sail when men fell from the rigging, but now the perineal portion of the urethra is more commonly injured by a hard kick in the crotch during a fight or while playing a sport. As it passes through the perineal wall just below the prostate, the urethra is very thin. The subsequent swelling and bruising worsens the damage, and if the urethra is very severely injured that portion may have to be removed and the urethra, rejoined. In all cases of injury to the urethra, strictures can occur long after the initial trauma and cause outflow obstruction. Occasionally the bladder and urethra are at risk from surgical and medical intervention. Although treatment of the bladder through the already existing opening of the urethra carries many advantages over open surgery, the procedures are fraught with hazards if carried out by inexperienced operators. Additionally, the presence of a resectoscope (an instrument for examining the bladder and removing tissue by electric current) in the urethra for the duration of an operation can result in incontinence afterward. Similarly, infection can be introduced into the bladder by a

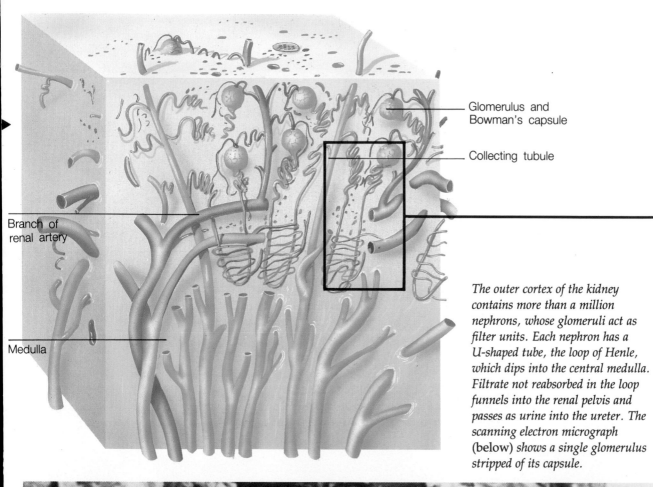

Glomerulus and
Bowman's capsule

Collecting tubule

Branch of
renal artery

Medulla

The outer cortex of the kidney
contains more than a million
nephrons, whose glomeruli act as
filter units. Each nephron has a
U-shaped tube, the loop of Henle,
which dips into the central medulla.
Filtrate not reabsorbed in the loop
funnels into the renal pelvis and
passes as urine into the ureter. The
scanning electron micrograph
(below) shows a single glomerulus
stripped of its capsule.

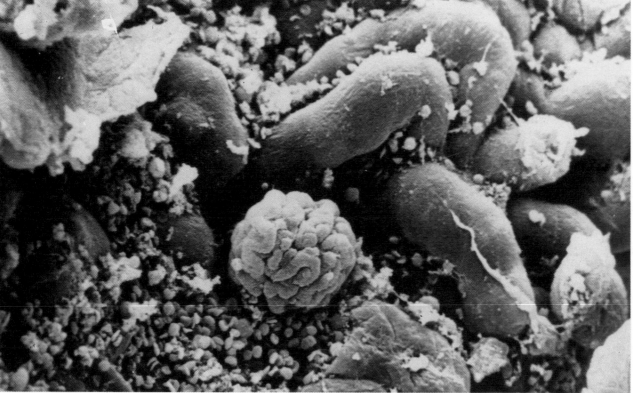

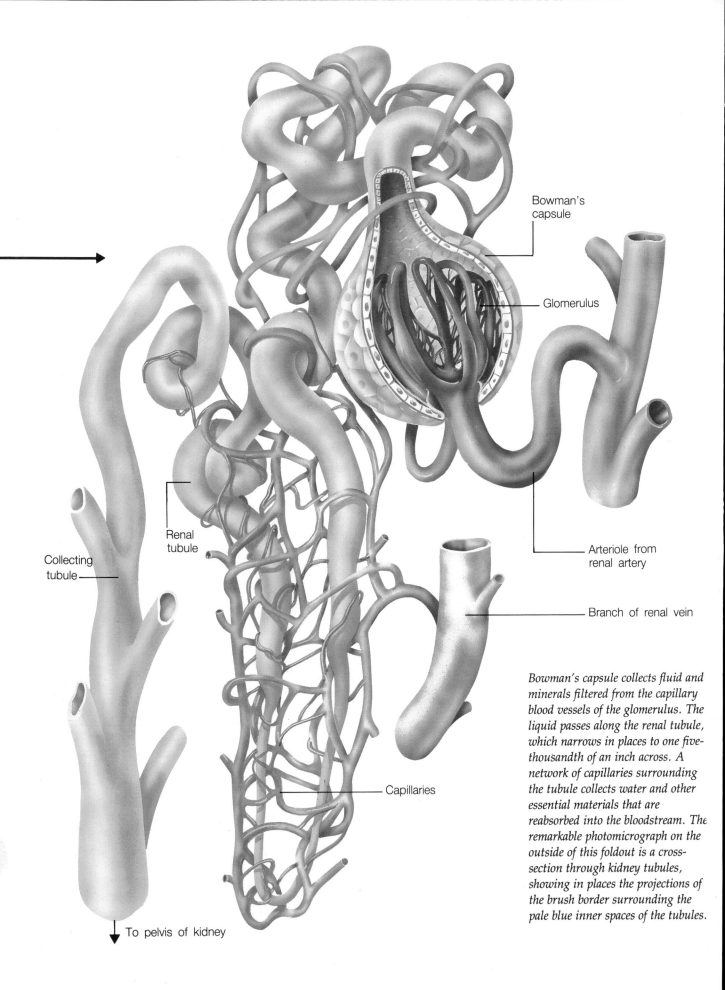

Bowman's
capsule

Glomerulus

Renal
tubule

Arteriole from
renal artery

Collecting
tubule

Branch of renal vein

Capillaries

To pelvis of kidney

Bowman's capsule collects fluid and
minerals filtered from the capillary
blood vessels of the glomerulus. The
liquid passes along the renal tubule,
which narrows in places to one five-
thousandth of an inch across. A
network of capillaries surrounding
the tubule collects water and other
essential materials that are
reabsorbed into the bloodstream. The
remarkable photomicrograph on the
outside of this foldout is a cross-
section through kidney tubules,
showing in places the projections of
the brush border surrounding the
pale blue inner spaces of the tubules.

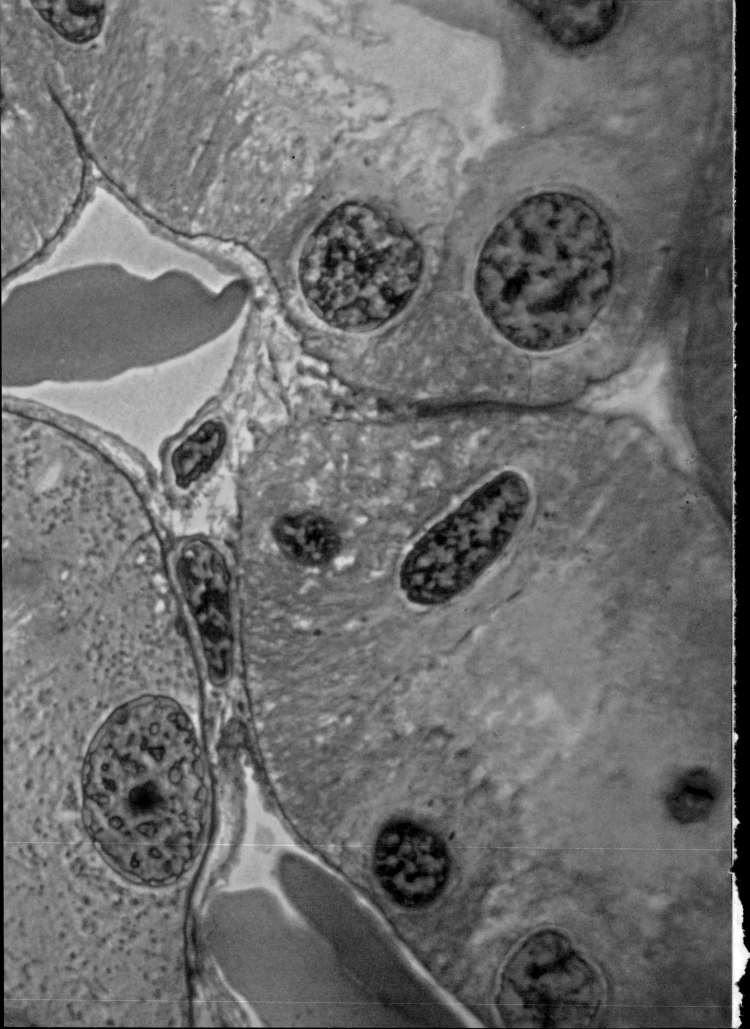

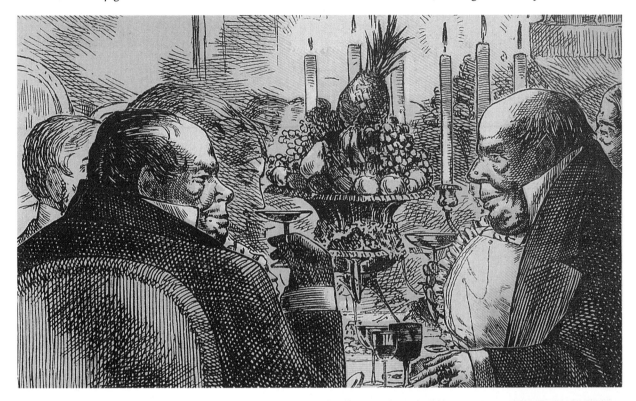

drainage catheter. However, with the development
of better instruments and techniques, there is less
chance of complications.

Removing Old Blood Cells

In addition to nitrogenous waste, there is another
by-product of metabolism which, although the
body can reuse a little of it, must eventually be
excreted. This is the hemoglobin from worn out red
blood cells.

A single organ is not responsible for this
breakdown in the way that the kidneys are solely
responsible for the production of urine. Instead, a
group of anatomically and geographically different
cells throughout the body deal with it. They are
known collectively as the reticulo-endothelial
system, and are found within the bone marrow, the
liver and the spleen.

Once broken down, the iron from the hemoglobin
is stored as ferratin for use later in the formation of
new cells, but the rest of the hemoglobin is
converted into the yellow pigment bilirubin and a
green pigment called biliverdin. The colors of these

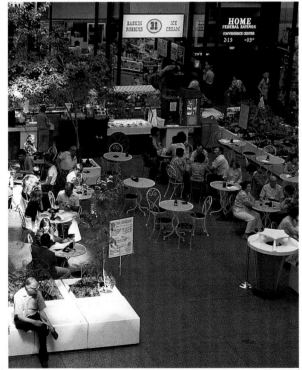

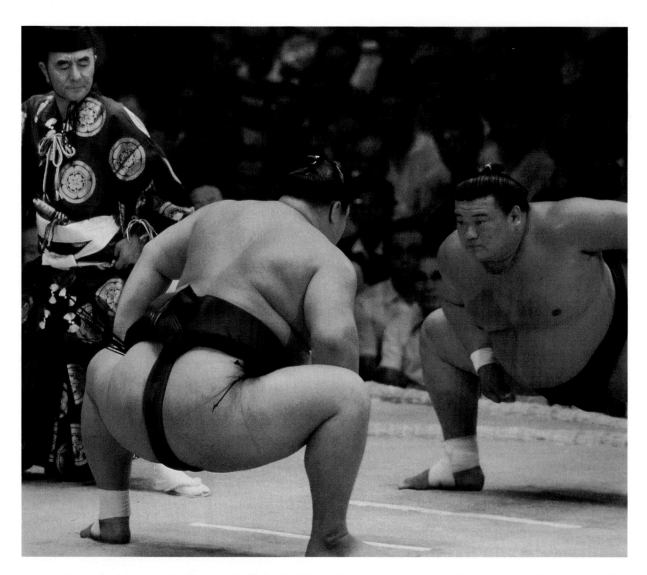

pigments can be seen as a bruise gradually heals. It begins as the blue-black color of reduced hemoglobin, then turns the color of biliverdin (which is green), and eventually changes to the yellow color of bilirubin. The body needs to rid itself of these pigments, but it can make one final use of them. They help to bring about the initial breakdown of fats and cholesterol during the process of digesting the food that has been swallowed.

Bilirubin and biliverdin are excreted as bile via the liver into the common bile duct and out into the duodenum. They pass on through the small and large intestines, where bacteria change the brown pigments into stercobilinogen and stercobilin, which give the feces their characteristic color. Any disruption of the excretory process of these pigments—for example, a gallstone lodged in the common bile duct — results in visible yellow pigment under the skin, the condition known as jaundice. In severe cases, little bilirubin passes to the intestines with the corresponding result that the feces are very pale.

Excreting Other Poisons

All drugs may be regarded as poisons, and most of them are actively excreted by the kidneys and liver. Drugs, particularly those that are in the blood plasma, pass through the walls of the capillaries in the glomerulus and into the nephron. From here they are washed away with the urea, but some drugs may be reabsorbed through the tubules (as are many of the components of urine). Doctors may administer other drugs to block active secretion into the kidney tubules, so increasing the activity time of the drug in the body in much the same way as drugs are used to block the reabsorption of uric acid from the kidneys in the treatment for gout. It is significant that the rate at which most drugs leave the system is directly related to the function rate of the kidneys, and a person with impaired function suffers drug overdose problems if given doses of drugs suitable for a person with correctly functioning kidneys.

Drugs that have a high molecular weight are usually excreted in the bile, although some may passively enter the system by diffusion and be excreted. Once the bile enters the intestines the drug may be altered or reabsorbed through the wall of the gut.

Volatile drugs — for example, those used during anesthesia — are excreted actively through the lungs. Acetone is a breakdown by-product of alcohol and because it is volatile can also be excreted by the lungs. The amount of acetone or alcohol in the breath can be measured and used as a test of drunkenness.

The body can also expel drugs through glands that are secretory in function, so that for a time these glands can be regarded as having an excretory role. They include tear glands, sweat glands and salivary glands, all of which can be regarded as a physiological oddity (rather than anything more serious). However, there is one set of secretory glands which can become excretory when drugs are in the body and have a detrimental effect — the milk glands in the breast of a nursing mother. Drugs enter the milk by passive diffusion, and a baby may become sleepy and unresponsive if the nursing mother is treated with drugs that suppress the central nervous system. Some types of antibiotics can come through the milk and cause discoloration of the child's secondary teeth (which are developing in the jaw of the baby). A potentially harmful extension of this principle is that antibiotics added to cattlefeed can be excreted in the milk of cows and cause allergies in human beings.

Kidneys are designed to keep the blood clean. Every minute of the day they filter out the impurities. But like any intricate structure, they have their limitations, and more and more they are having to deal with abuse. Some actresses, for instance, abuse their bodies by taking diuretic pills (to increase fluid loss) to maintain a body image they feel they should have in order to succeed. The kidneys are delicate organs that can be damaged not only by hazards within the environment but also by excessive taking of apparently harmless medicines such as aspirin or acetaminophen.

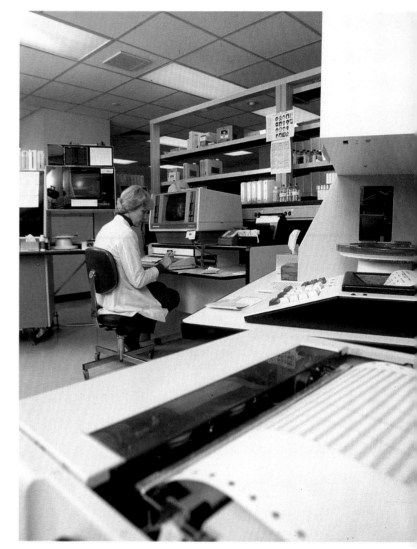

Certain malfunctions of the kidney can be detected by a urine test, which reveals, for example, the presence of proteins in the urine. In the pathology department of this American hospital, tests are rapidly evaluated using a computer linked to an autoanalyzer.

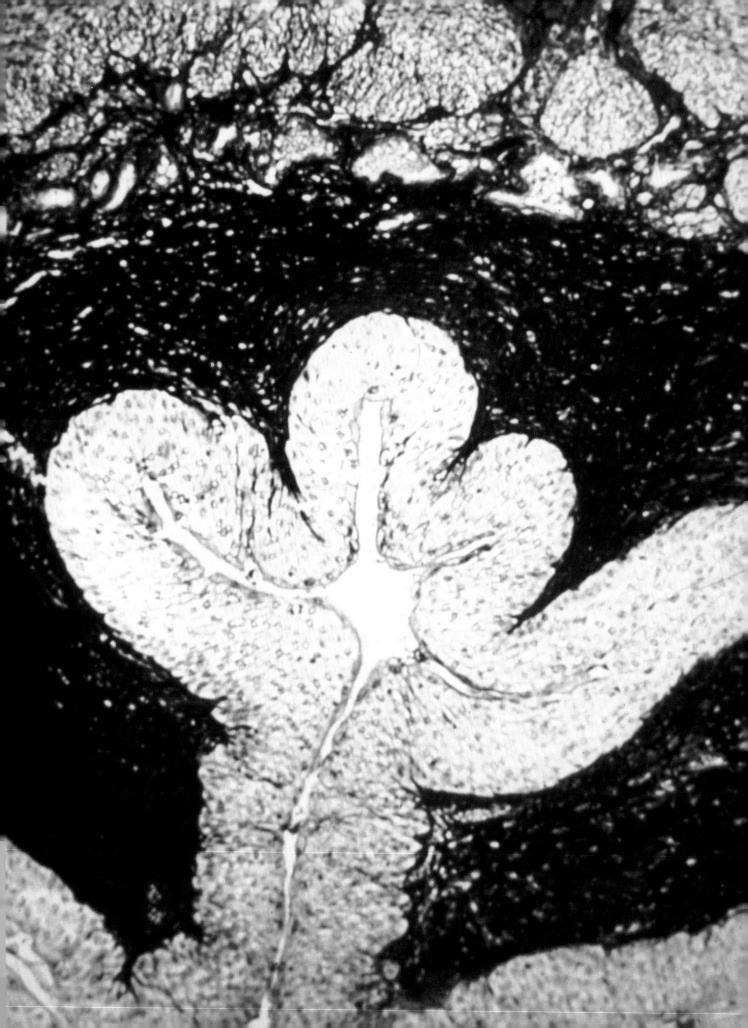

Chapter 3

The Balancing Act

Imagine a tiny single-celled organism floating about in the vast Pacific Ocean. For this minute creature, the environment in which it lives remains relatively constant — after all, a few rainstorms or showers over the ocean are hardly likely to dilute the sea, nor will evaporation of the water by the sun have any appreciable effect on the concentration of the salt it contains. So this cell lives in a stable environment and has no problems in getting rid of any waste products: they leave the organism and become infinitely diluted.

A single-celled organism, such as an ameba, living in a small freshwater pond faces a much more hostile and hazardous environment. A vigorous rainstorm may further dilute the already solute-poor water in the pond, causing water to enter into the body of the ameba by osmosis, the process by which water passes through a membrane separating solutions of different concentrations. If osmosis continued unchecked, the organism would swell and eventually burst. So special adaptations (contractile vacuoles) have evolved to eject any unwanted water in the animal cell.

On the other hand, if the pond begins to dry up during a drought, the concentration of dissolved substances in the pondwater increases, and water leaves the ameba, causing it to shrink. Again the cell has evolved a protective mechanism: it becomes encysted and surrounds itself with a waterproof coat to withstand dehydration. When weather conditions improve, it frees itself and becomes mobile again.

Warm-blooded multicellular animals have adapted to life on dry land by taking with them their own environment. All cells within the body are bathed in fluid, which enables them to exist in a relatively stable environment, despite wide variations in the outside world. It was the famous French physiologist Claude Bernard who, in the nineteenth century, first recognized the presence of this internal environment. He called it the *milieu intérieur* — what scientists now term the extra-

Only about one-eighth of an inch in diameter, the narrowness of the ureter — one of two tubes which carry urine from the kidney to the bladder — is revealed in a micrograph of a stained cross-section. Already one of the most well-researched organs in the body, the kidney still has some secrets to surrender.

Cells taken from the cheek appear as a cluster of islands in a green sea. The nineteenth-century French physiologist Claude Bernard was the first to identify what he called the milieu intérieur: "The true medium in which we live is neither air nor water but the fluid that bathes the tissues." The composition of this so-called interstitial fluid is largely controlled by the action of the kidneys.

John the Baptist (right) baptizes Christ by the Jordan River. The cleansing property of water is used in religious imagery to symbolize the washing away of sin and the purification of the soul.

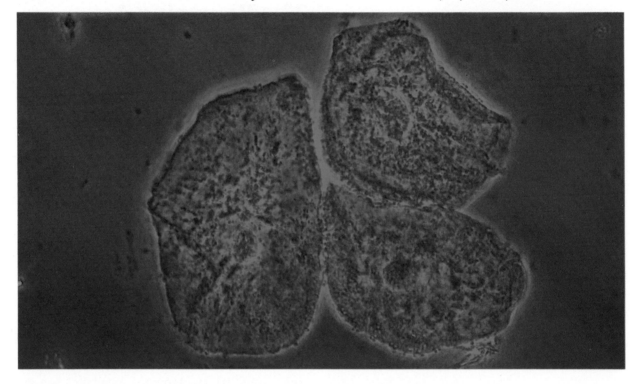

cellular fluid. Fluids inside cells are known as intracellular fluids.

Human beings therefore have two body-fluid compartments: the extracellular compartment which, in an adult, totals about twenty-five pints, and the intracellular compartment, which is about fifty-one pints. It is the careful regulation of the composition and volume of the extracellular fluids which provides a stable environment in which cells can exist. Through the extracellular fluid cells obtain nutrients and oxygen, and excrete their waste products. The only natural entry point to this internal environment is through the mouth, in the fluids and foods we drink and eat. In the small intestine, which is more than eight feet long, nutrients and vital salts are absorbed into the extracellular fluids. Most of the water is absorbed in the colon, which forms the greater part of the large intestine, just over three feet in length.

By contrast, there are four exit routes for extracellular fluid. One is through the skin, where a salty fluid is lost as perspiration, or sweat. The amount of fluid lost by this route depends on body temperature and the temperature and humidity of the surroundings. For example, if someone is sitting reading in a comfortable temperature of about 70°F, less than three fluid ounces of perspiration is lost each hour. But during strenuous exercise sweating is initiated, and a person can lose up to four pints of sweat each hour.

The evaporation of sweat helps the body to lose the extra heat it generates internally from the muscular work. If the environmental humidity is high, however, evaporation is severely reduced although sweating continues unabated. Strenuous physical work under such conditions could result in the body's losing up to eight pints of sweat an hour, but such rates can be maintained for only short periods. This is why living in the hot humid Mississippi basin may be far less comfortable than living in a drier environment at a much higher temperature on the equator.

The second route by which the body loses water is from the lungs, and this loss is related to the need to moisten the air that is breathed. In a dry climate more water is needed to moisten the air, and so more water is lost with each breath out. Thirdly, the body can lose abnormal amounts of fluid through

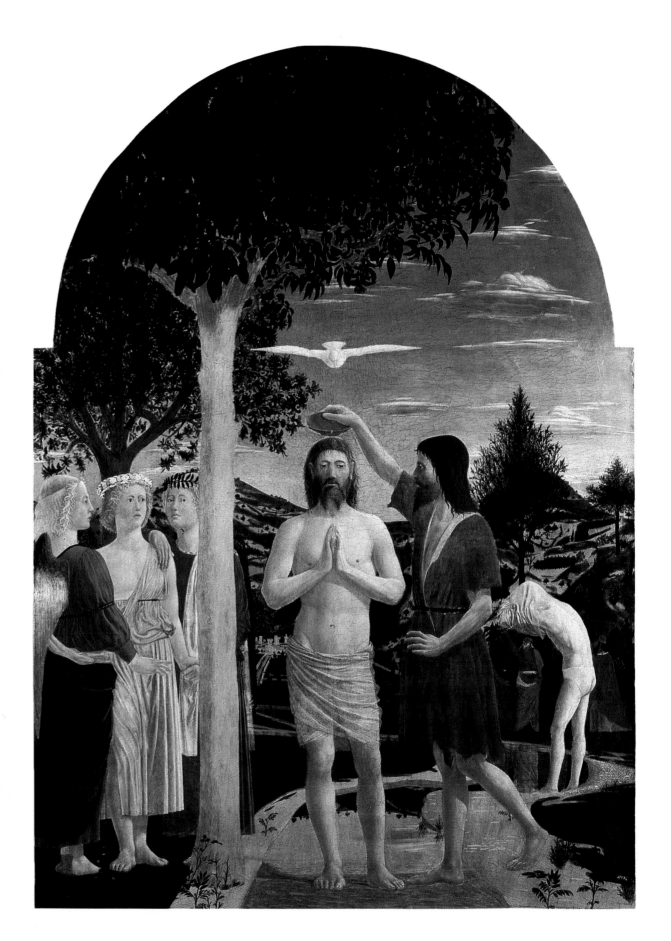

A staggering sixty per cent of our bodyweight is the water contained within cells and the medium in which they "swim." The mouth is the only natural entry point for this fluid, but we lose a daily average of

five pints in various ways. If there is excessive fluid loss the kidneys compensate by adjusting the production of urine. Strenuous work in humid climates can lead to the loss of eight pints of sweat an hour.

"Water, water, every where, nor any drop to drink": the stranded sailors in Coleridge's poem The Rime of the Ancient Mariner (right) *were unable to quench their thirst because salt water causes further dehydration.*

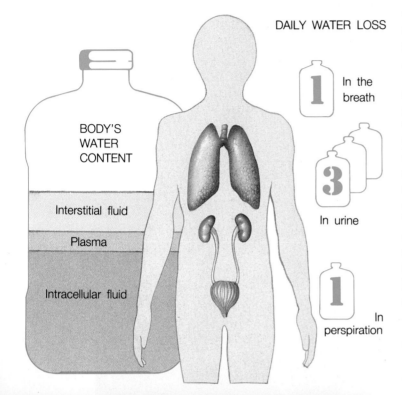

DAILY WATER LOSS

BODY'S WATER CONTENT

Interstitial fluid

Plasma

Intracellular fluid

1 In the breath

3 In urine

1 In perspiration

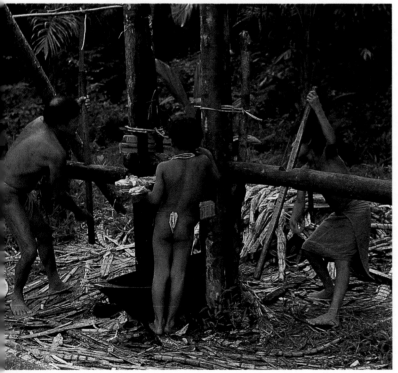

vomiting or diarrhea, when the gut fails to reabsorb the digestive juices it secretes or fails to absorb some or all of the water taken in as part of the diet. As a result, the body may become dehydrated.

The fourth and most important exit route of the extracellular fluid is via the kidneys: the organs, above all others, that control the composition and volume of the *milieu intérieur*. It is there that waste products of the extracellular fluid are excreted and the actual volume of extracellular fluid balanced by altering the amount of urine produced. It is there also that the pH (acidity or alkalinity) and salt content of the extracellular fluids can be regulated. Thus, it is only in the kidneys that the losses of the extracellular fluid can be controlled, and this is why these organs are essential for maintaining a stable internal environment. Their function is to act as a buffer against the potential hazards of a hostile and changing outside environment.

Compartments of the Extracellular Fluid

The extracellular fluid is more than merely liquid flowing about the body. It has precise functions to perform, and is of two kinds. The larger part of the extracellular fluid (about eighteen pints) is known as the interstitial fluid. This directly bathes each cell. The second compartment is the blood plasma, the straw-colored fluid in which the red and white blood cells are suspended. An adult human has about six pints of plasma (the other four pints of blood volume is occupied by blood cells). Because plasma circulates through the body, it acts as a bulk transporter of water and solutes in the extracellular fluid. It can also serve as a route for the rapid and even distribution of very small quantities of biologically active substances, such as hormones and drugs.

Fluid passes readily from the plasma to the interstitial fluid, and the composition of these two extracellular fluids is similar, although plasma contains a much higher concentration of protein and has more sodium than is found in the interstitial fluid. What the kidney does to regulate the extracellular fluid is to filter the plasma in the glomeruli of the nephrons. (There are about a million nephrons in each of our two kidneys.) As this fluid — the glomerular filtrate — passes down the bending and twisting tubes of the nephrons,

58

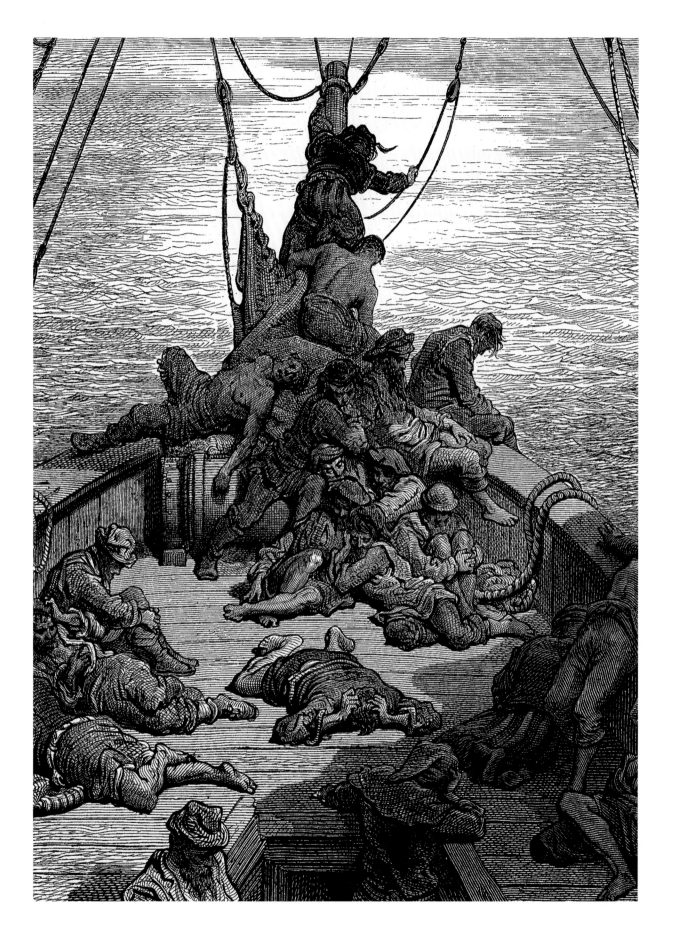

*The White Lady spider has adapted
to the arid conditions of the Namib
desert by getting all the fluid it needs
from the crickets that make up its
diet. South American lungfish
survive dry periods by tunneling*

*into the mud (right) until the return
of rains. In times of severe drought,
local people dig them out of their
habitat and squeeze the body fluid
out of the fish as a means of
obtaining water.*

*A street vendor (bottom left) sells
juice made from crushing split peas
—an unusual way of obtaining
fluids. As well as making a
refreshing drink, split peas provide a
valuable source of vitamins A and C.*

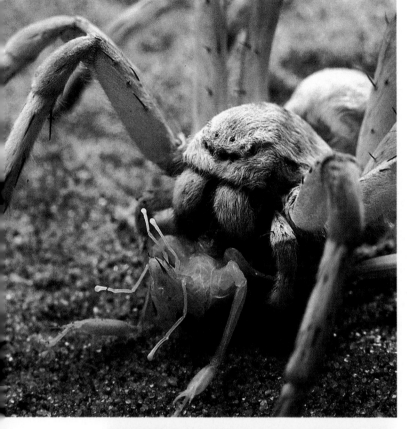

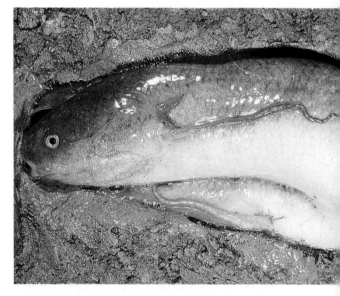

solutes and water are appropriately reabsorbed or allowed to be excreted in the urine, and in this way excess and waste products can be excreted while essential substances are retained within the body.

The Control of Body Water

In an adult, sixty per cent of the body weight is simply water, of which two-thirds is in the intracellular compartment, and one-third is in the extracellular fluid. In infants there is much more water (about seventy per cent by weight). The total amount of water in the body depends on the amount of fat — more fat, less water. So women, who have a relatively higher percentage of body fat than men, have proportionately less body water, whereas thinner people and infants have a proportionately higher water content, simply because their bodies contain less fat.

In normal circumstances everyone maintains a water balance, in that our intake equals our losses. Because we lose water with the moist air we breathe out, and because we perspire or sweat, the amount of urine produced is always less than our total water input. Everyone knows that thirsty feeling that follows hard exercise, hard breathing and profuse sweating. The body has become dehydrated, the extracellular fluid has been lost in the sweat, and more water than salts has been lost. As a result, the volume of the extracellular fluid is

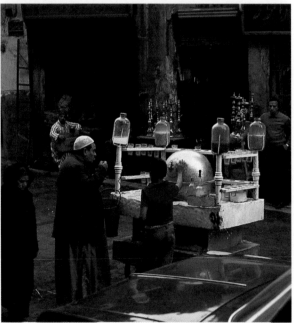

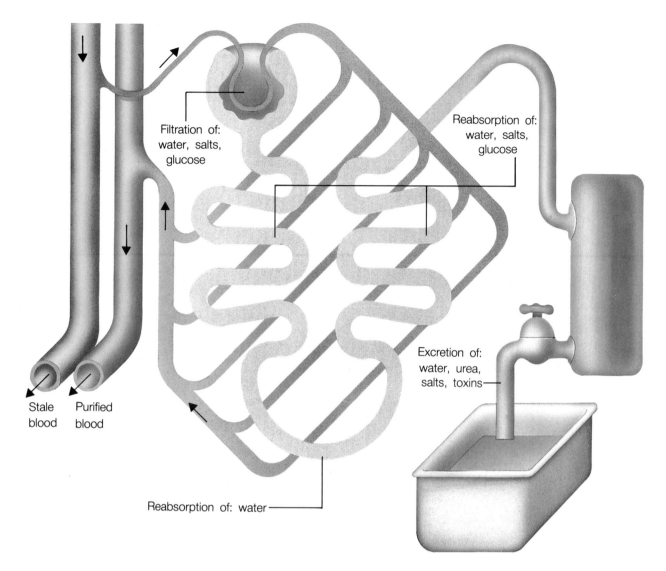

Filtration of:
water, salts,
glucose

Reabsorption of:
water, salts,
glucose

Excretion of:
water, urea,
salts, toxins

Stale
blood

Purified
blood

Reabsorption of: water

reduced and the salt concentration increased because of the disproportionate amount of water loss. We need to drink and we need to reduce the amount of fluid passed out in the urine. We feel thirsty, and a water-conserving mechanism in the kidney is switched on.

The amount of water passed out in the urine is controlled by antidiuretic hormone secreted by the pituitary gland. When the concentration of solutes in the extracellular fluid rises, as in dehydration, special cells in the brain detect the increased concentration (and hence osmotic pressure) of the fluid, and switch on the release of this hormone. The pituitary hormone gets into the circulation and so reaches the kidney, where it "instructs" it to reabsorb more water than normal.

In a normal day for the average adult, about three hundred and eighty pints of plasma are filtered through the glomeruli into the nephrons, and yet only about two to four pints of it appear as urine.

Within the pyramids of the kidney, millions of nephrons are responsible for purifying the body's blood supply and regulating the composition and volume of the urine. After the blood has been filtered in the glomeruli, fluid and essential products are reabsorbed from the tubules back into the surrounding network of capillaries. Of the 315 pints of filtrate produced each day, almost ninety-nine per cent is reabsorbed.

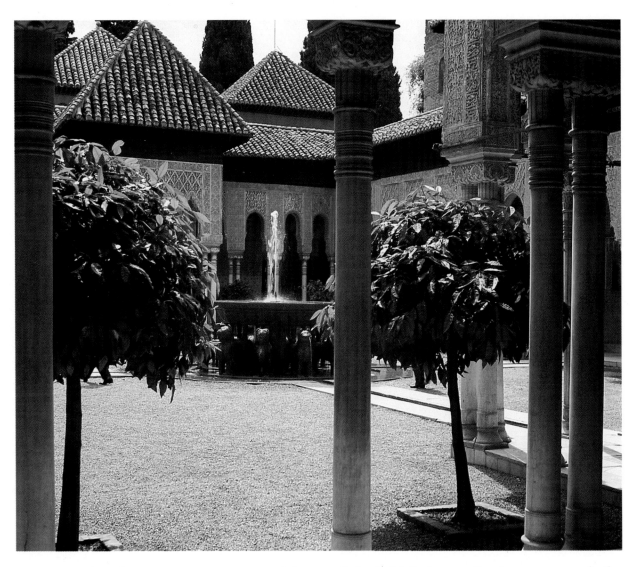

This means that about ninety-nine per cent of the filtered water is reabsorbed. A large proportion of it (up to two hundred and fifty pints) is "obligatory" water reabsorption, because it accompanies the reabsorption of sodium and chloride in the kidney tubules. As the salts are actively extracted from the filtrate in the nephron and replaced back into the extracellular fluid, water is "pulled back" into the body with the salt by a type of passive osmotic process.

Most of this type of "obligatory" water reabsorption goes on in the proximal tube of the nephron nearest the glomerulus. The structure of the loop of Henle, the distal tubule and the collecting ducts in the kidney enable urine to be produced. Urine can be more than four times as concentrated as the body fluids themselves (it looks a dark yellow color when this happens), or three times as dilute (almost colorless urine). This is because the loop of Henle can establish an osmotic gradient in the extra-cellular fluid that normally always surrounds the nephrons.

The osmotic concentration in the outer cortex of the kidney is low, but gradually increases as the middle or medullary part of the kidney is approached. Thus when fluid in collecting ducts passes from the cortex down toward the ureter, which emerges from the medullary region, water is again pulled out of the ducts by osmosis. This is where the antidiuretic hormone comes in. It opens up little pores in the collecting ducts. In this way more water is osmotically reabsorbed out of the duct back into the extracellular fluid, and water is conserved. It helps to compensate for any dehydration of the body and reduces the amount of water lost in the urine — so that the urine becomes very concentrated.

Of course, when we drink a lot of water our body fluids get diluted and then the release of anti-diuretic hormone is switched off. This means that

62

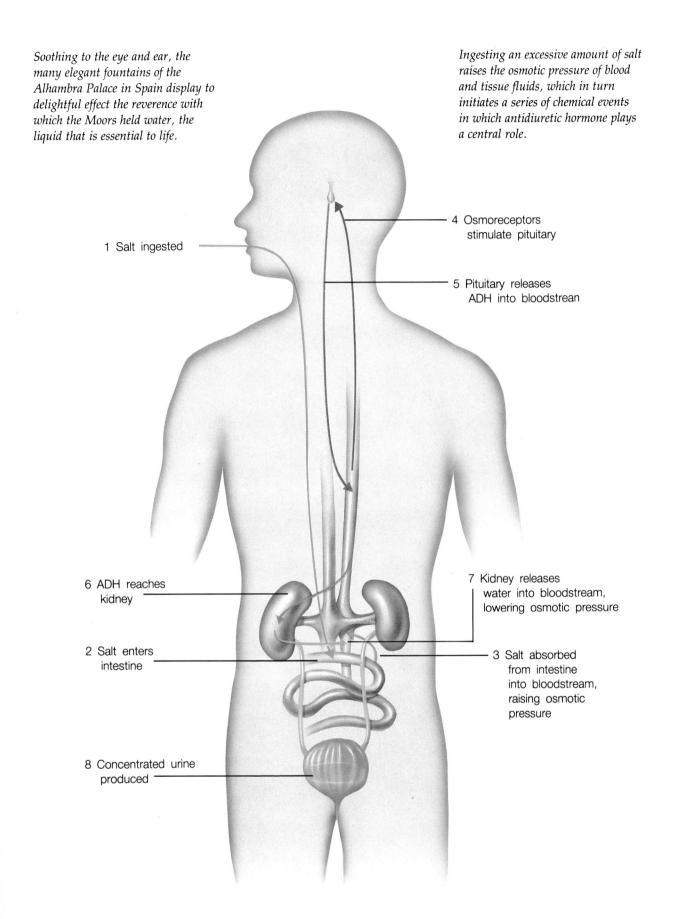

Soothing to the eye and ear, the many elegant fountains of the Alhambra Palace in Spain display to delightful effect the reverence with which the Moors held water, the liquid that is essential to life.

Ingesting an excessive amount of salt raises the osmotic pressure of blood and tissue fluids, which in turn initiates a series of chemical events in which antidiuretic hormone plays a central role.

1 Salt ingested

4 Osmoreceptors stimulate pituitary

5 Pituitary releases ADH into bloodstrean

6 ADH reaches kidney

7 Kidney releases water into bloodstream, lowering osmotic pressure

2 Salt enters intestine

3 Salt absorbed from intestine into bloodstream, raising osmotic pressure

8 Concentrated urine produced

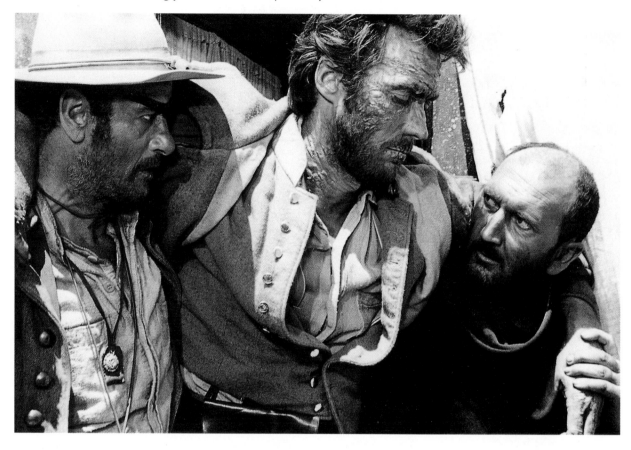

the collecting ducts are no longer very permeable to water, and so for a time copious amounts of dilute urine are produced.

The Regulation of Sodium

Sodium (Na^+), and its accompanying negatively-charged ions chloride (Cl^-) and bicarbonate (HCO_3^-), are in abundance in the extracellular fluid; none of the ions is present to any major extent inside the cells. If there is too much sodium in the extracellular fluid, water osmotically moves out of the cells to dilute the high salt concentration, and the cells become dehydrated. Conversely if the salt concentration falls, water moves into the cells and they swell. So the amount of sodium in the extracellular fluid does, to a large extent, determine the distribution of water between the extracellular and intracellular fluid compartments.

As soon as dietary salt — sodium chloride — is absorbed, it can be lost in sweat (and by diarrhea or

vomiting), but the kidneys are the only route by which the loss of sodium can be controlled. Sodium, along with chloride and bicarbonate, is filtered out in the glomeruli. About sixty-five to seventy per cent of this sodium is reabsorbed in the proximal tubule of each nephron, along with the "obligatory" water reabsorption. More of the sodium is reabsorbed in the loop of Henle, and most of the remaining sodium gets back into the extracellular fluid in the distal tubule.

In this part of the filter system the amount of sodium reabsorption is under the influence of the hormone aldosterone, but in fact the release of this chemical messenger is only the end point of a whole series of chemical events. The first part in the hormonal regulation of sodium reabsorption is the release of the enzyme renin from the walls of the blood vessels in the kidney when the flow through these vessels increases. Once released into the bloodstream, renin stimulates the conversion of a

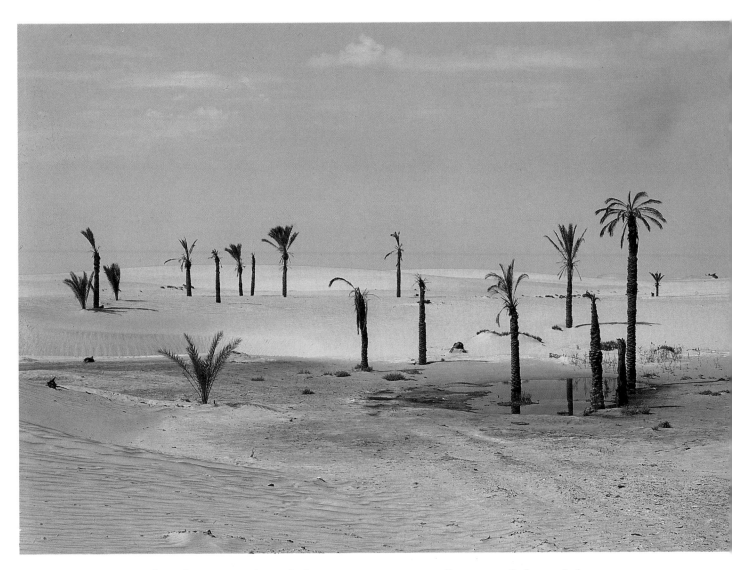

plasma substrate into the substance angiotensin I, which then undergoes a further chemical conversion in the blood to angiotensin II.

The hormone angiotensin II has two tasks to perform. Firstly, it acts on the two adrenal glands, which sit on the top of the kidneys. It causes the release of aldosterone from the outer cortex of the adrenals, and this hormone acts on the distal tubules in the kidney to increase the amount of sodium reabsorbed; in parallel, an increased amount of water follows. Secondly, angiotensin II helps to raise the blood pressure by increasing the resistance to blood flow.

The Kidneys and Blood Pressure

Two hormones — antidiuretic hormone (ADH) and aldosterone — can control the amount of water and sodium reabsorbed by the kidney, and both are involved in the long-term maintenance of normal blood pressure. It might seem strange that

On average, the human body can survive without water for up to seven days. Someone trekking across the desert, where temperatures can reach a scorching 100°F or more, and humidity is virtually zero, would need to find an oasis within half that period of time to stay alive.

Before it can be excreted, the sodium we consume must be diluted. Salty snacks may satisfy a temporary hunger pang, but lead also to a compensatory thirst — well satisfied, perhaps, by eating some juicy fruit.

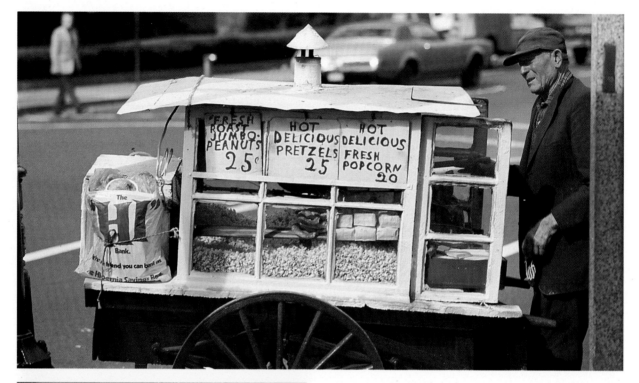

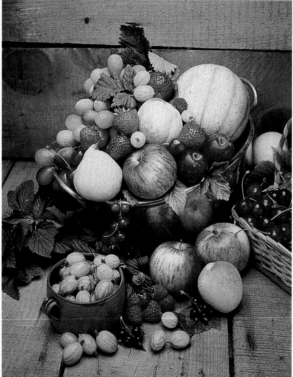

urine production is related to blood pressure, but the link between the two is shown by the following sequence of events.

In a sudden severe hemorrhage, the blood volume goes down and there is a precipitous drop in blood pressure. The immediate response of the body is to shut down many of the blood vessels, except those supplying vital organs such as the brain and heart, and to increase the rate of the pumping action of the heart. In the longer term, the body needs to restore the fluid loss of the extracellular fluid, and this is where the kidney plays a vital role. The low blood volume stimulates the release of antidiuretic hormone, which ensures that the maximum amount of water is reabsorbed back into the extracellular fluid. The low blood pressure also initiates the release of renin, and this increases the production of angiotensin II and so stimulates aldosterone secretion from the adrenal glands. More sodium and more water are pulled back into the system, and this helps replace the fluid loss and restore the blood pressure.

After a hemorrhage there is not only a loss of plasma volume, but also a loss of blood cells. Again, though, the body has evolved a mechanism by which it can compensate for the loss of red blood cells. When the red cell population decreases, as after a hemorrhage or in anemia, the manufacture of new red cells in the bone marrow increases. This effect is brought about by the hormone erythropoietin, which is formed from a plasma protein under the influence of a renal erythropoietic factor. In some way, therefore, the kidney senses a decrease in the red cell mass and releases the erythropoietic factor.

So what happens when the situation is reversed and the plasma volume expands or blood pressure is raised? The answer is that renin release is inhibited so that aldosterone secretion is reduced, and the release of antidiuretic hormone is also minimal. The net outcome is that less sodium and water are reabsorbed, and the body rids itself of extra fluid. This helps to lower the elevated blood pressure. This is also why people who suffer from hypertension may be placed on a low-salt diet. When there is not much salt in the body, very little renin and angiotensin II (which has blood-pressure raising effects) are free in the blood. Furthermore, if there is less salt to be reabsorbed, less water is reabsorbed and this again helps to keep the blood volume, hence pressure, in check.

Another substance that promotes the excretion of sodium has been found in the walls of the heart. When blood pressure rises, this "hormone" is released from the heart and inhibits sodium, and hence water, being reabsorbed from the kidney, thus causing a diuresis. Called the atrial natriuretic factor, it demonstrates a direct chemical link between the cardiovascular system and the excretory functions of the kidney, and confirms an old hypothesis that "another factor" controls the kidney's handling of body sodium.

Body Fluids in Abnormal States

It can happen that the regulatory system is stressed, and dietary salt and water supplies are not "balanced" by salt and water losses. Normally, in such a circumstance, the relative volumes of the extracellular to intracellular compartments is in the ratio of one-third to two-thirds and there is an osmotic balance between the two compartments. If a man is stranded in the Sahara at high noon, miles

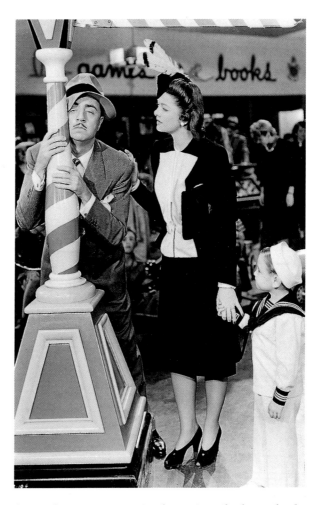

from the nearest oasis, he primarily loses body water and the salt concentration of his extracellular fluid increases. Although antidiuretic hormone may be gushing out from the pituitary gland, some water will still be lost in the urine and sweating continues unabated.

So as the concentration of the extracellular fluid increases, water moves out of the cells by osmosis and cellular dehydration results. The effects are most obviously seen as disturbances in the function of the brain cells — the poor victim goes "mad with thirst." At the same time, blood pressure falls, the pulse speeds up, the eyes sink into their sockets and the tongue becomes dry.

Now what happens if the situation is altered and the man finds himself on a raft in the Pacific Ocean. This is an example of the Ancient Mariner's observation "water, water every where, nor any drop to drink." In this case he is still exposed to sun and heat and he still has no fresh water — although surrounded by seawater. This has a much higher salt concentration than is ever found in the body, and is even higher than the most concentrated urine the kidney is capable of producing.

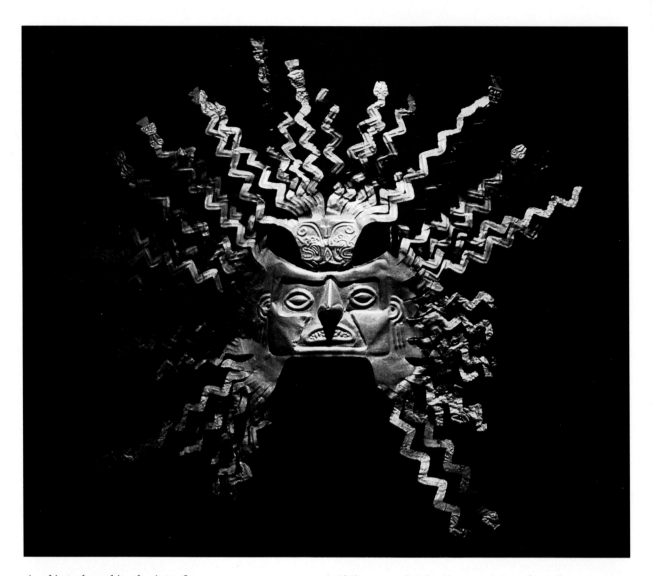

An object of worship, the Aztec Sun God stares balefully from the center of a gold mask. It is now known that sunlight is essential for health. It contains ultraviolet radiation which acts on the skin to synthesize vitamin D — the substance that promotes calcium reabsorption in the kidneys.

If the man drinks the seawater, the salt concentration of the extracellular fluid again goes up and so water moves out of the cell by osmosis, and the cells become dehydrated. Unfortunately, he could not even get rid of the salt in the urine without further depleting his body of water, because the salt would have to be diluted before the kidneys could excrete it. So the wretched person merely makes his situation worse by drinking the seawater, and would certainly suffer a more dramatic and rapid death than someone who has the willpower to resist the desire to drink.

These extreme examples illustrate the close link between sodium and water in determining the distribution of body fluids. In a normal healthy person, not enduring extremes in climate and situation, any excess of sodium ingested in the diet causes a thirst, and the subsequent compensatory drinking to dilute the body fluids expands the extracellular fluid. In time, the kidneys balance the equation. It is no accident that in some bars salted peanuts are provided free, because the thirst they produce may be profitable!

Drinking relatively large quantities of alcohol also causes dehydration, and results in the dry mouth and heavy head felt the morning after. Alcohol depresses the release of antidiuretic hormone and this causes a diuresis; more water than is appropriate is lost in the urine, and the body becomes dehydrated. For this reason, drinking a couple of large glasses of water after a party and before going to bed may help to offset some of the symptoms of a hangover.

People with heart disease may not be able to cope with an increased fluid load that follows drinking to compensate for eating salted peanuts or a salty meal. Blood volume goes up and excess fluid is forced out of the tiny blood vessels and into the interstitial fluid. This accumulation of interstitial fluid produces visible swelling called edema. Firm pressure on such a swollen area leaves an indentation, giving rise to the clinical sign of "pitting edema." This is another reason for people with heart failure and high blood pressure to be careful about their dietary salt intake.

Edema is, however, a general term which describes an expansion of the interstitial volume caused by sodium and water retention. It does not arise only in heart failure, and several other conditions — such as obstruction of a vein or lymph vessel, liver disease and renal failure — may also cause edema, albeit by somewhat different mechanisms. It is also common in pregnancy. The treatment is to administer diuretics — specific drugs which promote the loss of sodium and water in the urine — thereby alleviating the problems that result from having an expanded interstitial volume.

Balancing the Salts

On a normal North American protein-rich diet and with normal metabolic activity, the body is constantly producing hydrogen ions. The concentration of these ions is expressed as pH; a pH of 7 is neutral, less than 7 is acid, and more than 7 is alkaline. The pH of the extracellular fluid is usually 7.4 (slightly alkaline). In the events of everyday life, the variation of the extracellular pH is very slight.

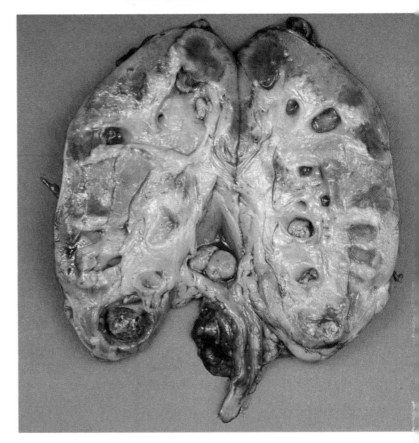

In decline in the temperate regions of the West, kidney stones — seen here embedded in a dissected kidney — are more common in hot climates, where sweating can concentrate calcium in the urine.

But in some profound pathological situations, the pH may be as low as 6.4 (acid) or as high as 7.7; beyond these limits survival is not normally possible, and the patient dies.

There are three available mechanisms for regulating changes in pH. Firstly, the body fluids contain buffers which can mop up the excess hydrogen ions and so prevent an increase in acidity (a decrease in pH). For example, if some hydrochloric acid were added to a bucket of water the pH of the liquid would drop rapidly. If the same amount of acid was infused into a dog with the same volume of water in its body as there is in the bucket, there would be little if any change in pH — the acid would be neutralized by blood buffers. These buffers provide an instantaneous mechanism to control pH, but in the longer term the lungs and the kidneys must get rid of any excess acid.

When the buffering systems become saturated, and the hydrogen ion concentration goes up, the

The key role of water — the ultimate necessity of life — is reflected in the religious beliefs of Hindus, to whom the Ganges River is sacred and, for pilgrims on its banks, has miraculous properties.

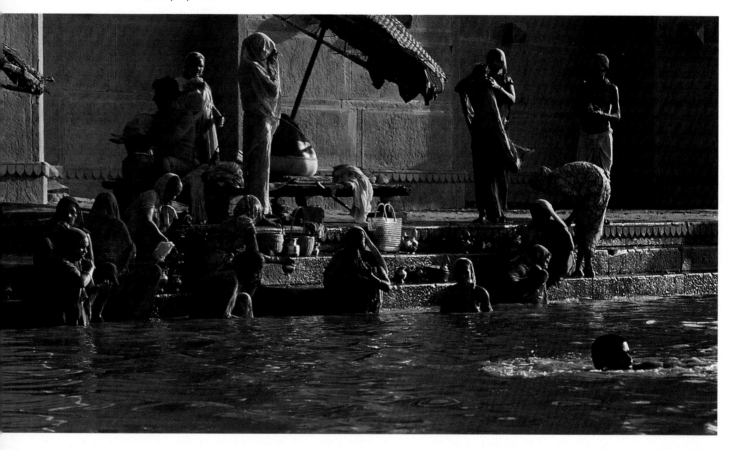

rate and depth of breathing may increase. This causes more of the waste gas carbon dioxide to be blown out of the lungs and, to maintain the chemical equilibrium, more carbon dioxide and water are formed from the bicarbonate (HCO_3^-) and hydrogen (H^+) ions in the blood. In effect this means that hydrogen ions can be turned into carbon dioxide (CO_2) and water (H_2O), and so the more carbon dioxide is breathed out, the lower the hydrogen ion concentration in the extracellular fluid becomes.

The renal response to changes in pH is the slowest, but is very important for the long-term maintenance of a stable pH. From carbon dioxide and water the cells of the kidney tubule make bicarbonate ions and hydrogen ions. The bicarbonate buffer is reabsorbed back into the body, and the hydrogen ions are excreted into the lumen of the tubule in exchange for sodium. For every hydrogen ion lost in the urine, a bicarbonate ion is retained, which is then available to neutralize or buffer further hydrogen ions in the extracellular fluid. In addition, the kidney can also excrete acid by the formation of ammonium ions (NH_4^+) from ammonia (NH_3), or through other buffers such as phosphate which can also "mop up" and excrete hydrogen ions.

The Kidney and Calcium

There are more than two pounds of calcium in the adult body, about ninety-nine per cent of which is stored in the bones of the skeleton. Calcium ions form complexes with phosphate, and the crystals of calcium and phosphate deposited in the skeleton make the bones rigid. The tiny amount of calcium floating around in the extracellular fluid is, however, extremely important because this ion has such profound and diverse effects within the body. It is a crucial component of muscle contraction (including heart muscle); it is important in

Homer Smith

Pioneer in Renal Research

Although he never had any formal training in medicine, Homer William Smith made a major contribution to the present-day understanding of the physiology and function of the kidneys. An author of both technical and popular works, he was responsible also for maintaining a prestigious laboratory.

Smith was born in January 1895 in Denver, Colorado. He was the youngest of his family's six children and, after attending high school at Cripple Creek, graduated from the University of Denver in 1917. World War I was still in progress, and his initial military experience was in a corps of engineers, but he then became a member of the Chemical Warfare Station of the American University in Washington DC. Accordingly, once hostilities were over he resumed his studies, this time at Johns Hopkins University, from which he received his doctorate in 1921.

Two years later he became a research fellow at Harvard, under the direction of Walter B. Cannon who (apart from his celebrated work on traumatic shock) was deeply interested in homeostasis — the regulation of the internal environment. Smith remained there for a further two years before he became Chairman of the

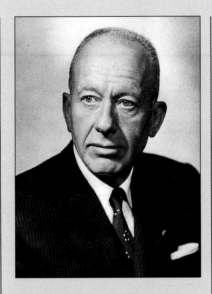

Physiology Department at the University of Virginia School of Medicine. And in 1928 he left again to take up the position of Professor of Physiology at the New York College of Medicine and Director of its laboratories. He remained there for the rest of his working life, during which time the laboratories became an internationally-acclaimed center for renal research.

It was following his period of study with Walter Cannon that Smith seems to have decided to specialize in research into the kidneys, their physiology and function. And having made the choice, he became probably the most knowledgeable person in the world on the subject — even to the extent of once describing the kidneys as "the

stuff of philosophy itself." It is evident that to him, homeostasis and the maintenance of what Claude Bernard called the *milieu intérieur* constituted not just a rich field of study in an area that had been neglected previously, but a fascinating theme by itself.

Yet initially, Smith began his investigations not into the kidneys of humans but into those of fish. He then proceeded to study seals and some land creatures. In pursuit of further information about mammals Smith took to spending the summers at the Mount Desert Island Biological Laboratory in Maine.

What seemed most fascinating to him was the process of filtration and collecting data for a comparison of blood flow rates. It was Smith who first understood much of what is now known about how the kidneys "clear" many individual constituents in blood — such as urea and sodium — and measured glomerular filtration rate (GFR). He also experimented with blood flow through normal and diseased kidneys, with special reference to high blood pressure.

He retired in 1961, to die a few months later, in March 1962, in New York.

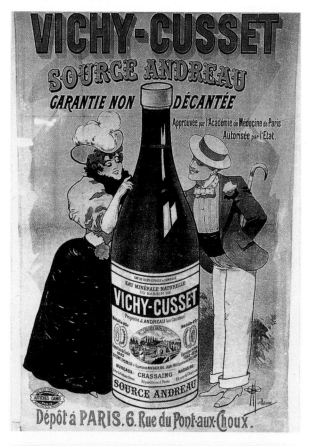

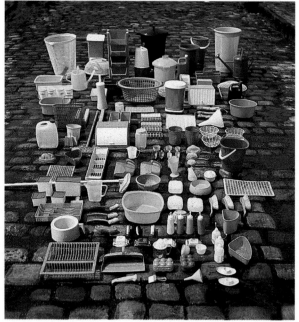

controlling the excitability of nerves; it is essential for the release of hormones and digestive enzymes; it acts in many metabolic processes; and it is part of the mechanism of blood clotting.

For these reasons, if the concentration of calcium in the extracellular fluid is not precisely regulated, small gains or losses of this ion may be critical to survival. When calcium is low, muscular spasms or tetany occur, with muscle cramps in the hands and feet; sometimes even convulsions are induced. In contrast, high levels of calcium can cause depression, problems in the digestive tract, calcification of soft tissue, and the formation of kidney stones because of the high concentration of calcium being excreted in the urine.

The extracellular fluid normally obtains calcium from the diet, although there are also stores of calcium in the bones. Calcium leaves the extracellular fluid either by being deposited back into bone or by being lost in the urine. Thus the kidney, as well as the gut and bone, is an important site for the control of extracellular calcium. Two major hormones are calcium regulators: parathyroid hormone (PTH) and vitamin D. Parathyroid hormone comes from the four parathyroid glands located on each of the four poles of the thyroid gland in the neck. When calcium levels in the extracellular fluid fall, PTH is secreted and the hormone helps to release calcium from bone (in the presence of vitamin D) and to increase the amount of calcium reabsorbed in the kidney; in parallel the excretion of phosphate is increased. These effects all help to restore depleted calcium levels in the extracellular fluid, and so PTH is said to have calcium-raising properties.

The action of vitamin D also helps to raise extracellular calcium by increasing calcium absorption in the intestine, promoting calcium reabsorption in the kidney and, in the presence of PTH, releasing bound calcium from bone. Our diets contain limited amounts of precursors of vitamin D, mainly in eggs and fish. The major source of this vitamin is, however, from the skin, where the action of ultraviolet light in sunshine converts precursors into vitamin D. This substance then has to be chemically changed before it is active in the gut, kidney and bone. The first step occurs through the action of a specific enzyme system in the liver

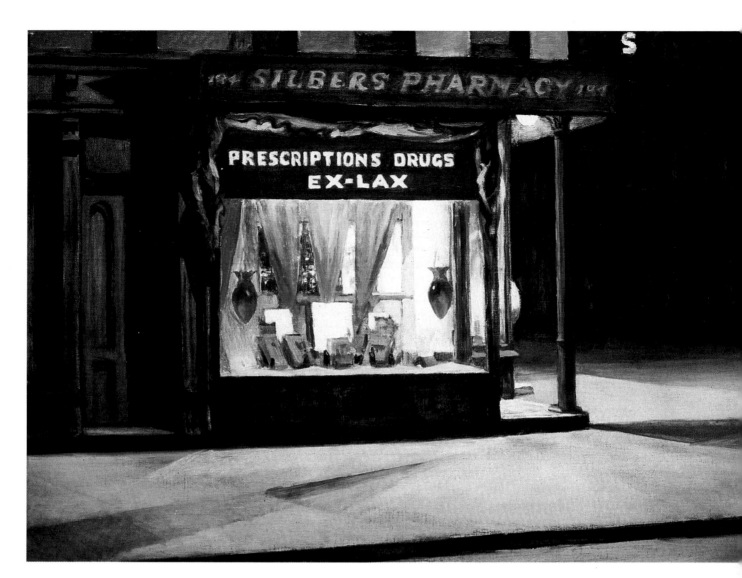

and the second in the kidney itself, helped by the action of PTH.

A deficiency of vitamin D in growing children produces rickets, a condition in which the skeleton is poorly calcified and the ends of the bones become swollen. Bowleg and knock-knee are the typical features of severe rickets. This bone disease was first described in the seventeenth century, but it was not until after World War II, when rickets became prevalent in Europe, that the relationship between calcification of bone, sunlight and vitamin D was understood, even though the concept of vitamins had been introduced at the turn of the twentieth century. In adults a lack of vitamin D produces osteomalacia, in which there is a loss of bone mass because calcium moves out of the bone.

The Kidney as an Excretory Organ

In addition to its role in controlling a stable composition, volume and distribution of body

Most drugs are filtered through the kidney, where the acid-alkali balance of the body largely determines their rate of excretion from the system. To avoid upsetting this delicate excretory mechanism, non-prescribed drugs should be taken with caution.

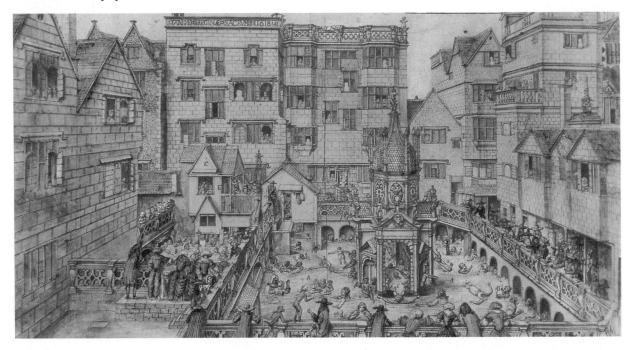

fluids, the kidney is also an important excretory organ for waste metabolic products released from cells, and for the excretion of hormones and drugs. Some waste products in the plasma are simply filtered through the glomerulus, and during the passage of the glomerulus filtrate through each nephron some part of the waste products may be reabsorbed, the rest appearing in the urine. On the other hand, some waste products may not be reabsorbed and all of the product filtered in the glomeruli appear in the urine. Certain drugs may not only be filtered in the glomeruli but are also actively secreted into the tubules from the rest of the blood flowing through the kidney. In this case, all the plasma flowing through the kidney may be cleared of a substance rather than simply the fraction of plasma which normally represents the glomerular filtrate.

One of the major excretory products is urea, which is the end nitrogen-containing product from the breakdown of proteins in the body. Urea is freely filtered in the glomeruli, but about one-half of the filtered substance is reabsorbed back into the bloodstream. Another waste product is creatinine, a breakdown product of phosphocreatinine, which provides a ''backup'' energy store in muscles. This substance is freely filtered in the kidney and is not reabsorbed. For this reason the amount of creatinine in the urine can be used as a clinical index of the glomerular filtration rate.

The removal of a hormone from the bloodstream after it has produced the desired effect on its target tissue is an important part of regulating endocrine mechanisms. Usually this takes place in two stages. The hormone is first inactivated or degraded, and then it is excreted. Some hormones are inactivated at the target tissue itself, some in the kidneys, but the most important site of hormone inactivation or degradation is in the liver. From there the ''treated'' hormones are either excreted in the bile, or passed back into the bloodstream and excreted through the kidneys.

The measurement of concentrations of hormones in the urine is often used clinically to assess the function of endocrine glands and to estimate the daily secretion rates of a particular hormone. For example, modern pregnancy tests rely on the detection of human chorionic gonadotropin in the urine of pregnant women, and the well-being of the fetoplacental unit during pregnancy can be determined by measuring the relative concentrations of estrogen and progesterone metabolites in the urine.

When penicillin was first introduced, grown as a mold (right), its production was costly and time-consuming. Urine from patients taking the antibiotic was saved, and the drug extracted from it.

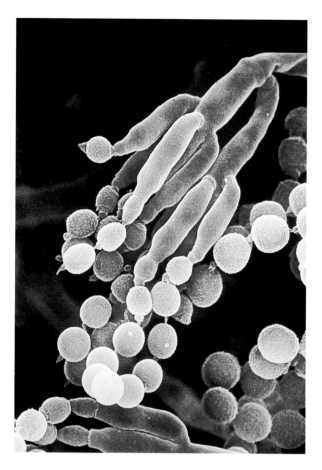

Most drugs are also excreted through the kidney, and the rate of their excretion depends to a large extent on the acid-alkali balance of the body. Generally, drugs are either weak acids or weak alkalies, and when they are absorbed into the body they exist in the blood plasma in a mixture of the ionized (charged) and un-ionized forms. Normally both forms of the drug are freely filtered in the kidney, but the ionized forms are not readily reabsorbed back into the blood whereas the un-ionized (uncharged) forms are lipid-soluble, and so readily pass out of the kidney tubules back into the extracellular fluid. Charged drug molecules are thus more rapidly excreted than the un-ionized form of drugs.

This property of drug excretion has been used to advantage to counteract the effects of drug poisoning. For example, in the case of an overdose of barbiturates (a weak acid), a bicarbonate buffer can be given to the victim, and this encourages the ionization of acids. As a result, more of the barbiturate drug in the kidney filtrate exists in an ionized form, and so less of the drug is reabsorbed. The consequence is that the drug is more rapidly eliminated from the body.

Some weakly acidic drugs are excreted very rapidly in the kidney. They are not only filtered in the glomeruli, but are also actively secreted into the lumen of the kidney tubule. Thus the blood flowing through the kidney may be nearly cleared of some drugs, including antibiotics, sulfa drugs and some diuretics. In fact when penicillin was first developed, the method of its production from microorganisms was both time-consuming and expensive. The urine from patients taking penicillin was "recycled" and the drug extracted from it. Today penicillin is often given in conjunction with another weak acid, probenecid, which competes with the drug for the active transport mechanism in the kidney. In this way less penicillin is actively transported from the blood into the kidney tubules, delaying its excretion.

It is thus easy to understand how kidney failure can lead to an abnormal build-up of metabolic products, hormones and drugs within the body, and how any impairment of their excretion alters their concentration in the extracellular fluid. A physician prescribing drugs to a patient with renal failure takes great care with the type of drug chosen and its dosage.

There are other substances which are freely filtered in the kidney but are required by the body. Glucose is the most notable, and for this reason all the glucose which is filtered is completely reabsorbed back into the bloodstream; none of it normally appears in the urine. Patients with untreated diabetes mellitus have high concentrations of blood glucose because they have no insulin to allow cells to take up the glucose from the blood. As a result the filtered plasma in the kidney contains so much of this sugar that the tubules simply cannot cope with the reabsorption. There is glucose in the urine, and this causes the sweetness of urine in untreated diabetics (hence the term *mellitus*, meaning "like honey"). The presence of the glucose also means that less water can be absorbed in the kidney, and so the volume of urine is increased (giving rise to the term *diabetes*, which means "one who is constantly passing").

There is another form of diabetes, called diabetes insipidus, in which there is a copious production of dilute or "insipid" urine. The condition has nothing to do with insulin and blood glucose, but arises when an individual does not produce anti-

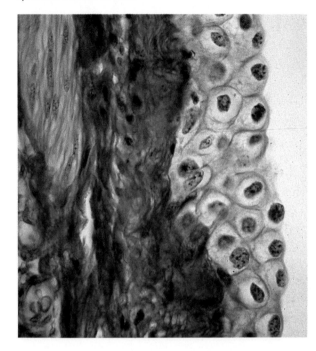

diuretic hormone. Consequently, very little water is reabsorbed in the collecting ducts and the body loses large amounts of water in the urine; the patient suffers continuous and intense thirst. Fortunately there is a drug which acts much like antidiuretic hormone but is more resistant to being degraded in the body, and this is used to treat patients suffering from diabetes insipidus.

The Urinary Bladder

The plasma is filtered through the glomeruli and, on its passage through the nephron, substances have been reabsorbed or secreted. Finally the modified filtrate reaches the ureters — the tubes leading from the kidney to the urinary bladder. The walls of the ureters are lined with smooth muscle which contracts at regular intervals — about one to five times a minute; spurts of urine are regularly ejected into the bladder. As the bladder becomes full the pressure within it rises, and when it contains about a pint of urine there is a great desire to urinate. Even when the bladder holds only about one-third to one-half a pint of fluid, a sensation of a "full bladder" may be felt.

Micturition, or urination, involves the reflex contraction of the detrusor muscle of the bladder,

and a relaxation of the sphincters in the neck of the bladder. These effects are brought about by the parasympathetic and sympathetic nerves of the autonomic nervous system. Micturition can, however, be consciously suppressed until a socially convenient time and place. The autonomic parasympathetic reflex for micturition can thus be inhibited, and relaxation of the bladder and contraction of the sphincters can be voluntarily initiated. Micturition is held in abeyance until there is a conscious relaxation of the sphincters, contraction of the bladder and an increase in abdominal pressure caused by a voluntary contraction of abdominal muscles. In normal circumstances, then, micturition is a complex response to the bladder filling and is under both voluntary and involuntary (parasympathetic/sympathetic) control.

Sometimes when someone gets very cold or is severely stressed, the muscular tone in the bladder wall increases so that a critical pressure within the organ is reached even though a maximal capacity of the bladder has not been achieved. This is why people often "feel" that their bladders are full and that they need to micturate when stepping out into a cold environment. It also explains why a sudden shock or very stressful situation may cause inappropriate urination. The bladder contracts, the pressure builds up and without the control of conscious faculties the bladder empties by an unconscious reflex. The bladder sphincter and urethra also receive a nervous innervation from the sympathetic branch of the autonomic nervous system. It is thought to cause contraction in the smooth muscle in these regions and so prevent the possibility of semen refluxing back into the bladder in males.

Any damage to the nerves controlling the bladder may lead either to urinary incontinence or urinary retention with "overflow," depending on the precise site of the neural lesion. For example, in paraplegic patients with transections of the spinal cord, the conscious control of micturition may be lost although the reflex control can remain intact. They therefore have no means of voluntarily regulating micturition but some patients can train themselves to micturate by pinching or stroking their thighs. This provokes a mild mass reflex, part

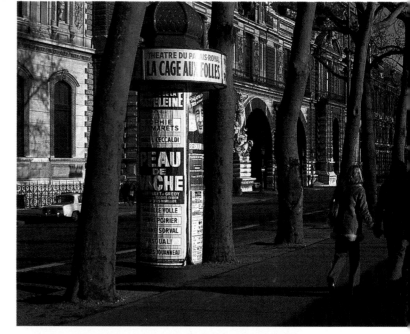

A call of nature can be answered in Paris by stepping into one of the numerous pissoires around the city (below right). They also provide a handy site for posters advertising the city's entertainments.

Bringing urination under conscious control so that the bladder does not empty automatically when full becomes second nature once learned, but is one of the more demanding tasks for a toddler (bottom).

of which involves the parasympathetic reflex of bladder emptying.

As already described, a common cause of abnormal micturition in adult males is an enlarged prostate gland, which can obstruct the outflow or urine from the bladder through the urethra. It is a problem which is particularly prevalent in older men, and normally surgical removal of the gland is undertaken, or the urethra is widened where it passes through the prostrate. Neither operation affects libido.

A further example of abnormal micturition may be found in pregnant women, when the high levels of progesterone may limit the degree of bladder control because the hormone tends to reduce the contractile "tone" in smooth muscle. Thus bladder emptying is impaired, and the sphincter control of urine outflow is reduced. This hormonal effect of progesterone may be distinguished from the purely physical effects caused by the growing fetus pressing down on the bladder.

Drugs that Affect Kidney Function

A group of drugs used therapeutically to alter kidney function are the diuretics, which increase the volume of urine produced. The most important are those which affect the excretion of ions such as sodium and hydrogen. These diuretics are used in treating edema, high blood pressure, and other related clinical states.

A second group of diuretics are those that effect water excretion. Alcohol is one such drug and its action on inhibiting ADH release and thus preventing water reabsorption has already been described. There are also several "osmotic" diuretics. They are inert substances which are freely filtered into the tubule and increase the osmotic pressure of the glomerular filtrate. This, in effect, limits the amount of water that can be reabsorbed. In general, though, this second group of diuretics is of little importance therapeutically.

A widely-used class of diuretics are the thiazides. Chemically they are organic compounds containing sulfur and nitrogen, closely related to the antibacterial sulfa drugs, and their diuretic effects were in fact discovered accidentally in the search for antibiotic agents. What thiazides do is to inhibit the active reabsorption of sodium in the distal tubule of

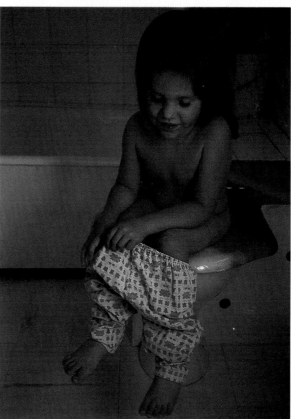

Urine—normally a waste product —has a number of surprising applications. The Dinka tribesmen of the Sudan use the natural bleaching properties of cow's urine to lighten their hair.

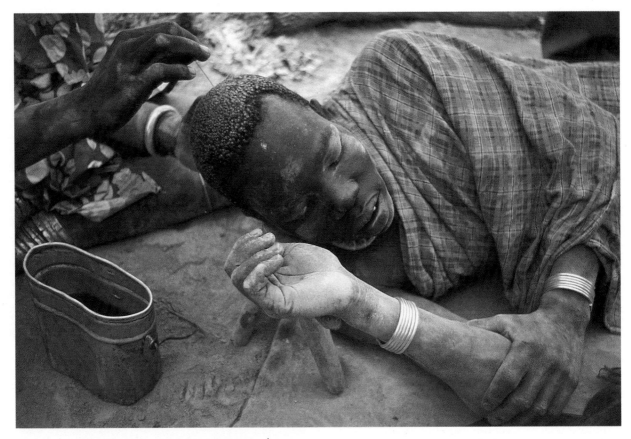

the nephron, and so less water is reabsorbed. The problem with these drugs is that they also increase the amount of potassium excretion, and depletion of potassium in the extracellular fluid can give rise to severe muscle weakness and abnormal rhythms of the heartbeat. However, these diuretics may be used in conjunction with an antagonist of aldosterone called spironalactone, which helps to limit the loss of potassium. The drug is thus defined as a potassium-sparing diuretic.

The other type of diuretics widely used is the loop diuretics, so called because they act on the loop of Henle. Their effect is to prevent the maintenance of an osmotic gradient from the cortex to the medulla and so, when the fluid in the collecting ducts passes down through these regions to the ureters, water cannot be osmotically reabsorbed. The drugs effectively make the kidney insensitive to antidiuretic hormone and so increase the volume of urine produced.

Loop diuretics are sometimes referred to as "high-ceiling" diuretics because, in contrast to the other classes of drugs, they produce a rapid and intense diuresis. When injected intravenously they act within minutes and can increase urine flow up to about forty milliliters per minute (the normal rate is about one to two milliliters per minute). Such an intense diuresis can produce an effect rather like that of a hemorrhage and so these drugs have to be used with extreme care.

One of the major clinical uses of diuretics is in the treatment of edema associated with congestive heart failure, cirrhosis of the liver, and chronic nephrosis in the kidney. In congestive heart failure, the blood cannot be pumped out of the heart fast enough so the pressure builds up in the veins returning to the heart. This "back pressure" eventually increases the capillary pressure, so more fluid is pushed out of the vessels and accumulates in the interstitial spaces.

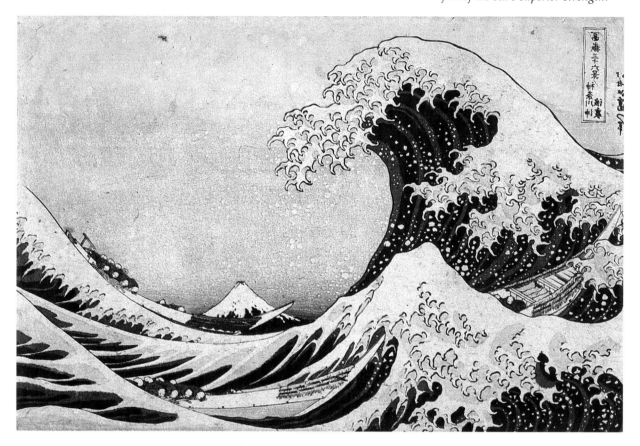

Another important clinical application of diuretics in the treatment cardiovascular disease is the use of thiazides in the treatment of patients with high blood pressure. These drugs are usually given in conjunction with another antihypertensive drug which has a direct effect on the pumping action of the heart. Edema also occurs when there is a loss of proteins in the plasma, either because the liver fails to make them or because large amounts are leaked across damaged glomeruli and are lost in the urine. Fewer plasma proteins cause the osmotic pressure of the plasma to be lower than normal, and so the osmotic force which pulls fluid back into the capillaries from the interstitium is reduced — fluid accumulates in the interstitial spaces.

Sifting, Saving and Excreting

The kidneys have the vital role of disposing of wastes and maintaining fluid balance. The American physician Homer Smith wrote: "It is no exaggeration to say that the composition of the body fluids is determined not by what the mouth takes in but by what the kidneys keep." He also pondered on the intricacies and sophistication of kidney function when he asked the question "What engineer would design an excretory system that throws everything out sixteen times a day and snatches back those things that it wanted to keep?" The unique structural properties of the glomeruli, through which three hundred and eighty pints of plasma are filtered each day, and the special reabsorptive and secretory transportation mechanisms in the kidney tubule, enable the blood plasma — and hence interstitial fluid — to be maintained within precisely-defined limits of composition and volume. Diseases may impair this careful balancing act between excretion and reabsorption in the kidney, but luckily modern dialysis machines and renal transplant surgery can redress the imbalances which result from kidney failure.

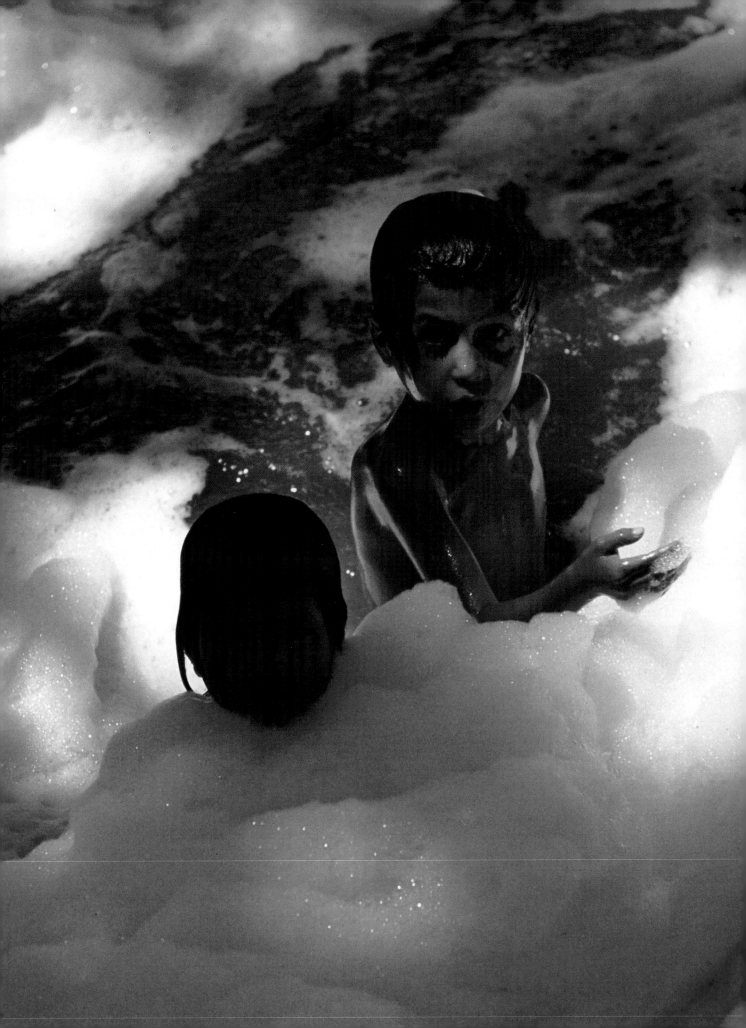

Chapter 4

Diseases and Disorders

The correct functioning of the kidneys is essential to physical well-being, and yet it is something most people take for granted. This complacency is perfectly understandable, firstly because of the comparative rarity of something going seriously wrong with the kidneys, and secondly because the condition of the kidneys does not usually feature in everyday conversation as other medical conditions may do. Yet, every year, thirty-five thousand people in the United States die from renal disorders, not including those who die from renal cancers. This figure is low compared with the annual total of seventy-five thousand deaths caused by heart disease, for example, but there are many more people who suffer from some episodes of renal and urinary tract problems at some time in their lives. And although such problems are often relatively minor and transient illnesses, they can cause considerable discomfort for the individuals affected.

It is estimated that twenty per cent of all women suffer one or more attacks of urinary tract infection at some time, and one per cent of the population develops a renal stone. Although the problem caused by such a stone is commonly a single episode, the associated pain can be excruciating, and for many patients represents the worst that they ever experience.

Despite the low overall death rate for kidney disease, many people suffer permanent damage to their kidneys, which therefore cannot function normally. It is for this group of people that there is a nationwide program of dialysis and transplantation, costing about two billion dollars every year.

Types of Kidney Disorders

Some kidney disorders occur in an individual for no known reason. Others, such as the condition known as polycystic kidneys, are hereditary and passed from one generation to the next in a predictable way. Such congenital disorders also include a horseshoe kidney, so named because of

Completely unaware of the risk of infection and the danger of ingesting toxic chemicals, these children play in Colombia's Bogotá River which is heavily polluted with industrial and organic wastes. The human body is well equipped to deal with its own wastes, but it is unable to neutralize and dispose of some of today's chemicals, many of which can cause kidney failure or other disorders.

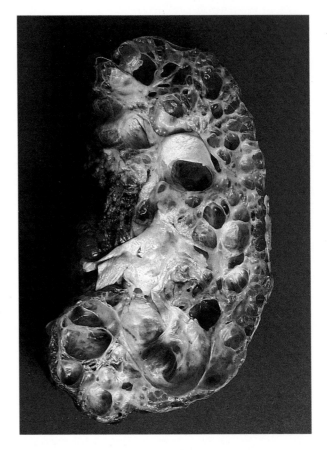

the shape formed by the two kidneys which are fused together, usually at the lower ends. Although the function of this kidney may be as good as normal, it gives a strange and characteristic appearance on an X ray.

Because the structure of the kidney is complex there are many things that can go wrong as the kidney develops in a fetus; disorders of kidney development are referred to as dysplasias. Extensive defects may give rise to early renal failure or stillbirth. Minor conditions, such as doubling of the renal arteries or of the ureters, are common and symptomless, and are recognized only as a chance finding later in life.

Kidney disorders may be acute (sudden) or chronic (long-lasting). For example, a renal stone may be an isolated event in the medical history of a particular individual, whereas some types of glomerulonephritis rapidly and relentlessly progress until the kidneys fail completely, and the only alternative is dialysis or transplantation. Other disorders — such as high blood pressure (hypertension) — may be chronic, but with early diagnosis and treatment their progression can be controlled.

Some disorders affect different age groups, such as the conditions that affect children mentioned earlier. The effects of disorders such as hypertension and diabetes mellitus usually take many years to become apparent, and so renal damage from these causes is more common among the elderly population. One severe form of the kidney disorder glomerulonephritis called Goodpasture's syndrome, by contrast, frequently affects men in their twenties and thirties.

Kidney disorders also vary in incidence from country to country. Sometimes this is related to common local infections such as malaria. In Egypt the parasitic disorder schistosomiasis, or bilharzia, is common, and one form of it infects the bladder. The condition predisposes the patient to bladder stones and to squamous carcinoma (cancer) of the bladder, which can result from severe and repeated inflammation.

Differences in incidence of kidney disorders between countries may sometimes alternatively be explained by cultural or industrial causes. Analgesic nephropathy is a condition that causes damage to the tubules and renal papillae, and is itself caused by abuse of painkilling drugs, especially those containing phenacetin. Total consumption has to exceed two pounds of the drug, equivalent to six tablets a day for four or five years. Many women take such drugs in quantity to relieve anxiety or depression, and the condition therefore tends to affect more women than men. The estimated consumption of phenacetin is four times higher in Australia than it is in the United States — and in Australia analgesic nephropathy accounts for about one-third of all the cases of chronic renal failure.

Exposure to harmful industrial chemicals can also produce diseases of the kidney and urinary tract. Naphthylamine was widely used in the rubber and plastics industry until health statistics suggested an association with tumors of the bladder. It took a long time to detect because the tumors did not appear until ten or even twenty years after exposure. Moreover, because the

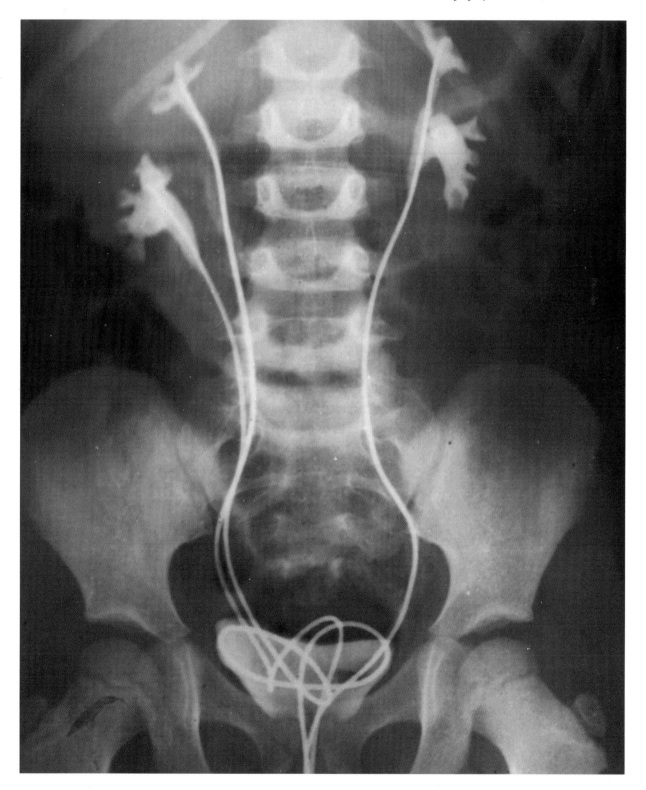

Triple ureters — in which one kidney empties into a double renal pelvis through paired ureters to the bladder — is a chance occurrence and does not normally cause malfunction or any symptoms.

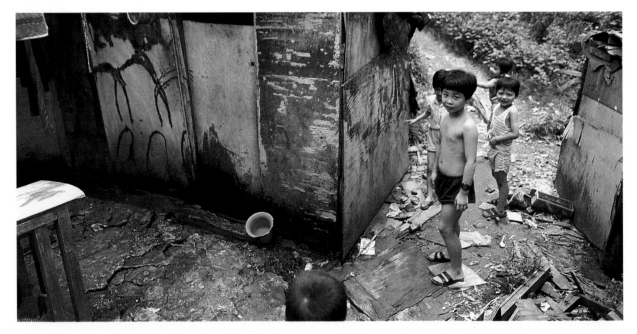

workers had often also changed jobs and moved to a different town, it was difficult to establish a link between cases. Naphthylamine has now been banned from use in industry.

Often, the first sign of a kidney disorder to be noticed by the patient is an abnormality in the coloration of the urine, sometimes combined with increased or reduced frequency of urination.

Abnormal Urine

Hematuria, or the appearance of blood in the urine, is a symptom that usually causes alarm. Bright red urine is not, however, always a sign of bleeding. The coloration may be caused by the excretion of some harmless but highly-pigmented compound, as may occur for instance after eating red beets. If there is actually blood in the urine it may be detected by a simple test carried out by the family physician who may then be able to diagnose it as being produced by any one of a variety of disorders. Common causes are certain conditions of the lower urinary tract, such as infections, a stone or even a bladder tumor, but diseases of the kidney, such as glomerulonephritis, polycystic kidneys or a renal tumor may all cause blood to leak into the urine. The amount of blood that appears in the urine varies from only a few red blood cells, which goes

unnoticed by the patient and can be detected only by microscopic examination, to such a severe loss that the urine seems to be entirely of blood. Only a few drops of blood are required in a pint of urine to cause a noticeable color change.

Proteinuria, or the presence of protein in the urine, is another common symptom of renal disease, but is generally invisible to the patient. Again it can be detected quite simply by the family physician or hospital laboratory. Most of the protein is albumin, and so the condition is commonly also called albuminuria. Between one and five per cent of the population of the United States are found to have proteinuria on routine testing — an unexpectedly high proportion. For most, however, it is a benign condition caused by some poorly understood change in renal hemodynamics, leading to proteinuria in otherwise normal individuals. In these people protein is found only in urine formed while they are in the standing position, and not in the urine formed when they are lying down, a condition termed orthostatic proteinuria. Proteinuria is also one of the main early symptoms of hypertension in pregnancy. It may additionally be a symptom of glomerulonephritis and similar disorders.

If the protein loss is severe, the osmotic pressure

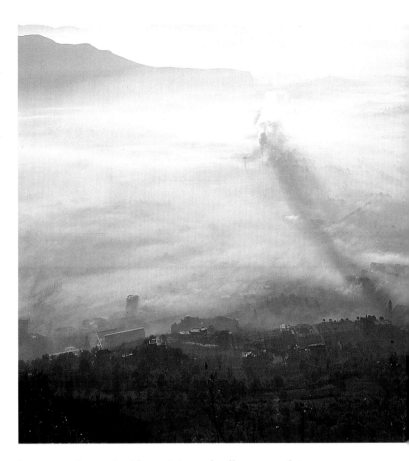

of the circulating blood falls, and as a result fluid passes out of the blood into the tissues. The tissues swell with fluid and the patient develops a puffy appearance, particularly of the face. The swollen extremities and puffy features of edema, or dropsy as it was once called, have been recognized for hundreds of years, and as early as the thirteenth century a connection with the kidneys was made by the Italian surgeon William of Saliceto. The precise cause of dropsy was not determined, however, until the nineteenth century, when the British physician Richard Bright made a study of the pathology of the kidney and its association with edema. Proteinuria is sometimes referred to as Bright's disease, in recognition of his work.

Loss of more than one-sixth of an ounce of protein in the urine per day, leading to edema, is termed the nephrotic syndrome. As fluid leaves the blood, the circulating volume falls, resulting in compensatory urinary salt and water retention. This causes further dilution of the blood and worsens the problem, as a vicious circle develops.

Inflammatory Disorders

Glomerulonephritis, or inflammation of the glomeruli, is associated with various disorders and accounts for thirty per cent of cases of chronic renal failure. A small number of cases are now preventable, and others respond well to early treatment. Diagnosis is aided by the removal of tiny pieces of tissue under local anesthetic to carry out a renal biopsy, which can provide vital clues to the state of the kidney.

In most cases, however, the exact cause remains a mystery, although antibodies in the blood are known to be involved. These highly specific proteins home in on and bind to a target (antigen) in the kidney. As the glomeruli become damaged, cells proliferate and fill the blood spaces, and with time the glomeruli become scarred and useless. Sometimes a thick layer of protein is laid down over the walls of the blood vessels in the glomerulus (membranous glomerulonephritis), which clog up and become scarred.

In Goodpasture's syndrome, the circulating blood somehow contains an antibody to the basement membrane of the glomerulus. As more and more antibody sticks to it, the glomerulus becomes clogged with protein and cells accumulate in Bowman's space to form a characteristic crescent. The lungs are also affected, and the patient may cough blood. The root of the disorder thus seems to lie within the bloodstream, and some patients therefore have the plasma fraction of the blood removed using a special machine and replaced with fresh plasma. Plasma exchange, or plasmaphoresis as this process is called, allows the patient to keep his or her own red blood cells, but to take in clean plasma containing no antibodies. The procedure has to be repeated as more antibody builds up, but is a useful treatment.

Sometimes the antibody formed is specific to something in the blood itself, such as another protein or an infective agent. When this happens, the antibody and the other agent bind together as immune complexes which, on reaching the kidney, can become trapped — partly because of their large size and surface charge — and cause inflammation. This occurs in rheumatoid arthritis, cancers and infections such as malaria, producing membranous glomerulonephritis.

Infections caused by some strains of *Streptococcus* bacteria, which cause sore throats and scarlet fever, sometimes lead to glomerulonephritis which occurs a few weeks after the initial infection,

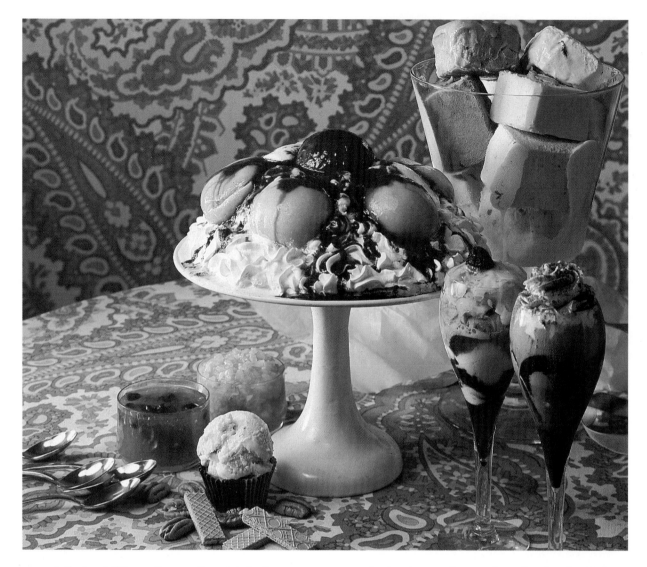

especially in children. Severe throat infections are much less common since the introduction of modern antibiotics and improved standards of hygiene and living conditions.

If, in addition to proteinuria, the glomerular disease is severe enough to cause a sudden increase in blood pressure and hematuria, the disease is termed acute nephritis. Children who develop the nephrotic syndrome or nephritis usually make a full recovery; adults do less well, however, and may develop acute or chronic renal failure. There are also many other patterns of glomerulonephritis which may produce the nephrotic syndrome, hematuria, proteinuria or renal failure.

Urinary Tract Infections

Infections of the urinary tract are a common problem and, except in the first few months of life, occur much more frequently in females than males. The reason for this difference is that females have

a much shorter urethra — the tube that leads from the bladder to the outside — which provides an easy route of infection from the exterior. Foreign bodies such as stones or tumors may also precipitate infection. Outward signs of bladder or kidney infection may be few — or be represented in a number of symptoms.

An infection of the bladder makes passing urine painful, and patients often describe a burning sensation. It also becomes difficult to start the stream although there is an urge to pass urine very frequently. The symptoms are collectively referred to as cystitis. If a clean specimen of urine is obtained without contamination from skin cells or vaginal organisms (called a midstream specimen), it can be cultured in the laboratory to identify the cause of infection, which is usually one of the bacteria normally found in the bowel.

In some people, bacteria can be found in the bladder but there are no symptoms; this is called

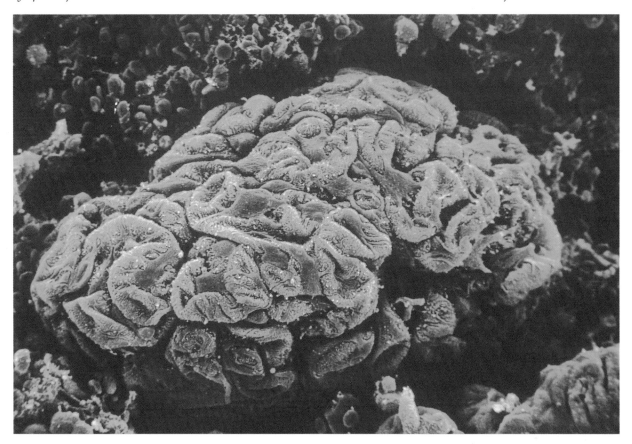

asymptomatic bacteriuria. In others, no cause can be found or there is inflammation in adjacent (paraurethral) tissue, and this is termed the urethral syndrome. Tight underclothes and personal deodorants may contribute to the condition. A catheter provides a direct route for the entry of infective organisms, and bladder infection is common in catheterized patients. Untreated bladder infection may very occasionally spread back up the ureters to the kidney and cause pyelonephritis.

In women, symptoms of infection are sometimes associated with sexual intercourse — "honeymoon cystitis" is a common condition. A high standard of personal hygiene and drinking plenty of non-alcoholic fluids help to prevent recurrent infections (because urination automatically flushes out any new bacteria introduced into the bladder). Treatment of the first attack is usually straightforward, and a single dose (or short course) of antibiotics is all that is required. If infection recurs, the bacteria may become resistant to the drugs used or a new, more virulent, strain may take over. Some patients require long-term courses of antibiotics.

Sometimes at the lower end of the ureters the mechanism that prevents urine from the bladder traveling back up to the kidneys is faulty, a condition known as "reflux." Such a backflow can damage the kidney in either or both of two ways. There may be increased pressure within the renal pelvis because of the flood of urine passing backward from the bladder. These parts of the kidney may then become distended and be permanently damaged. Alternatively, the urine which is refluxing may be infected, and so introduce infection to the kidney; this gives rise to acute pyelonephritis. Reflux may be present in babies and young children; surgery is not ordinarily required — but if the problem is recognized late, at say the age of five years or after, the kidneys may

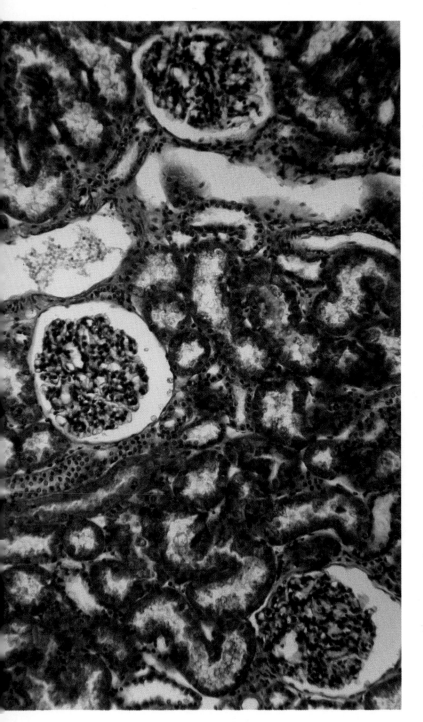

The crescent-shaped areas of this micrograph are the result of Goodpasture's syndrome, in which the kidney's glomeruli become clogged with protein; cells then build up and distort the shape of the Bowman's capsules, which are normally spheroid.

be permanently damaged and hydronephrotic (distended). It is important to give treatment for any underlying cause of the infection, such as stress or reflux, especially in children, in whom permanent scars occur early in the disease.

Urinary infections are common in pregnancy, as is asymptomatic bacteriuria. Screening of urine samples is a routine part of prenatal care, because acute pyelonephritis is more likely to develop at that time. Acute pyelonephritis is infection of the pelvis and tubules of the kidney. In addition to pregnancy and obstruction, diabetes and immuno-suppressive drugs may be predisposing factors. There is usually fever, hematuria and shivering attacks (rigors). If the infection is untreated, abscesses form in the kidney and permanent scarring results. Even normally, the papillae of the kidney usually have a poor blood supply, and if it is jeopardized by infection, diabetes or analgesic abuse, the papillae may die and drop off in the urine (papillary necrosis).

Infection of the kidney is only one factor involved in the development of chronic pyelonephritis, and most patients also have obstruction or reflux. Unlike the acute infections, there may be no specific symptoms and the condition is revealed only during routine health screening, although some patients suffer from high blood pressure or general malaise. Chronic pyelonephritis accounts for twenty per cent of cases of chronic renal failure.

In men, infection of the prostate gland (prostatitis) may be acute or chronic, and is usually caused by the same bacteria from the bowel as those that cause urinary infections. Surgical procedures or catheterization predispose a patient to prostatitis. There may be backache, fever and pain on passing urine. Antibiotics are usually effective in treating the infection.

Sexually transmitted diseases are a common cause of inflammation of the urethra (urethritis). These disorders are divided into gonococcal and non-gonococcal urethritis (non-specific urethritis, or NSU). Some cases of NSU have no known cause, although microorganisms of the genus *Chlamydia* are responsible for about two-thirds of cases. The symptoms of all types of NSU are similar, with urethral discharge and pain on passing urine. The diagnosis is confirmed by examining a smear of the

Peter B. Medawar

Investigations into Immunity

Tissue rejection following a surgical graft or transplant from another person is one of the most common hazards of that kind of repair to the human body. The body's immune system simply will not accept any tissue that it distinguishes as foreign to itself. Evidently, to be able to overcome the problem—even to avoid it altogether—a considerable amount of information must first be gathered on how immunity arises initially, before birth. For his important work in this field, Peter Brian Medawar was awarded the 1960 Nobel Prize in Physiology and Medicine.

Medawar was born of British parents in Rio de Janeiro, Brazil, in February 1915. But it was from Magdalen College, Oxford, that he graduated in 1939, becoming a Fellow of the College at the same time. Concentrating on research into the blood clotting mechanism, he managed during the 1940s to derive a solution of the main clotting agent fibrinogen powerful enough to be used as a sort of adhesive fixative in the repair of nerves and the immobilization of nerve grafts. This was a particularly important field at the time— many burns patients were treated during World War II— but it also aroused Medawar's interest in the problems of

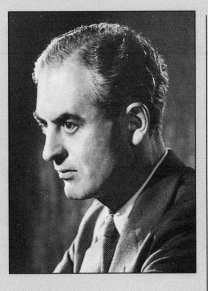

tissue rejection.

In 1947 he accepted the Chair in zoology at Birmingham University (in the English Midlands), although his doctorate was actually not to come through until the next year. He then transferred four years later to a similar post at University College, London. His appointment to the directorship of London's National Institute for Medical Research came in 1962, and a further senior post at the Clinical Research Centre from 1971 saw him to semi-retirement in 1975.

Medawar's initial research indicated that tissue grafting was normally successful not only between identical twins but also between fraternal twins. This suggested to

Medawar's colleague and mentor, the Australian-born immunologist Frank Macfarlane Burnet, that not just twins but *everybody*—early enough in the womb—might start with much the same kind of tissue, to which antibodies and other elements of the immune system were gradually added through individual circumstances, conferring an immunity system specific to each person well before birth. The problem was then to discover by experiment a time at which tissue was generalized in this way. Burnet's main thesis concluded with the rider that, if he was right, an embryo inoculated with foreign tissue at the appropriately early stage would not reject tissue from the same donor after birth.

This is what Medawar's research succeeded in confirming. He used two types of mice: one embryonic type was inoculated with tissue from the other; at that early stage no antibodies formed. At a later stage, when antibodies were capable of being formed in the mice, the experiment was repeated: again no antibodies formed. The ability of an animal to create specific antibodies was thus proved not to be inherited but to be developed individually by the animal after a certain stage of growth in the womb.

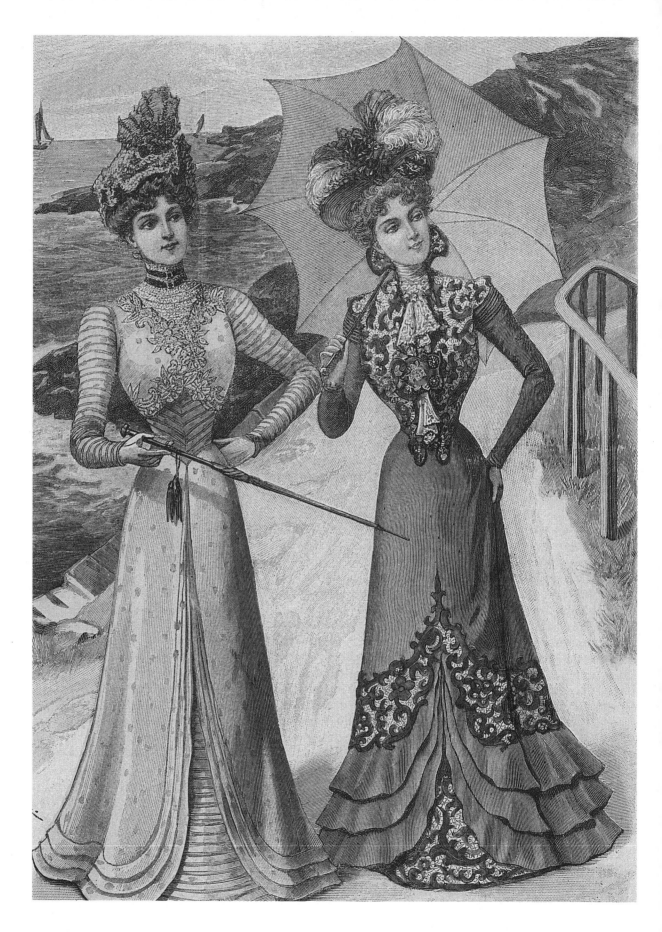

discharge in the laboratory and culturing it. NSU frequently responds to treatment with erythromycin or tetracycline. It is important that patients with a known venereal disease are carefully investigated for other sexually transmitted diseases, because multiple infection is common. Gonorrhea responds to high-dose penicillin, often administered as a single intramuscular dose, although the number of strains which are resistant to penicillin is increasing and other drugs may need to be used.

Tuberculosis affecting the renal tract is now extremely uncommon, partly because it follows lung infection, which is now treated promptly with effective drugs. But once the infection has taken hold, it may spread to the prostate and epididymis (in males), the bladder and the ureters. If the disease remains untreated, the kidney may be completely replaced by a mass of calcium and debris of a similar consistency to bone. The symptoms arising from tuberculosis are similar to those following other renal infections, and the tubercular bacteria can be detected in the urine. Identical drugs are employed to treat urinary tuberculosis and tuberculosis of the lung.

Urinary Tract Obstruction

There are many different causes of urinary tract obstruction, which can occur at any site from the renal calyces to the urethra. In children congenital abnormalities are a common cause, whereas in elderly men enlargement of the prostate gland is a common cause of blockage in the urine flow. Renal stones and tumors, especially of the bladder, are the other common causes. Sometimes a blood clot, pressure from a mass outside the urinary tract, or a faulty nerve supply may alternatively result in obstruction. On rare occasions infections such as gonorrhea and tuberculosis produce strictures of the urethra and ureter, reducing the tract to a passage so narrow as to obstruct the flow.

Because the urine flow is impeded, pressure builds up in the kidney and renal pelvis, and the ureters start to dilate. Eventually the kidney becomes swollen and the nephrons are damaged. In some cases the obstruction resolves without damage to the kidney as with most renal stones and blood clots, which are passed in the urine within a few days. In other cases, however, the obstruction does not resolve without medical intervention. This may involve ultrasonic treatment to crush the stone and flush it away, or surgery to remove a stone that completely blocks a kidney, or to remove a mass of bladder tumor that blocks a ureter as it enters the bladder. Rarely the obstruction cannot be adequately removed, and diversion of the urine is required. At one time a popular operation involved implanting the ureters into the colon, to allow urine to drain from the kidneys, but this is not a common procedure now because of the likelihood of infection and because of the disturbances to the mineral and acid balance which result. The urine may instead be drained directly to the exterior of the abdominal wall, or collected in an artificial bladder and then drained through the abdominal wall, in the same way as a colostomy.

Stones in the Kidney

Renal stones, or calculi, are common and are the cause of about one in every thousand hospitalizations in the United States. They are an old problem — stones have been found in Egyptian mummies. Some patients have a family history of stones and there are rare stones caused by hereditary metabolic defects. Considerable advances have been made in the surgical treatment of stones in the last ten to twenty years.

More than eighty per cent of stones contain calcium, usually as calcium oxalate; the rest contain phosphates or urates (as are formed in gout). If the concentration of calcium in the urine increases, stones are more likely to form. This may be caused by an increase in calcium circulating in the blood (hypercalcemia), an increase in calcium escaping in the urine (hypercalcuria), or both. Overactivity of the parathyroid glands in the neck, erosion of bone by cancer and dietary defects such as excessive milk intake or vitamin D overload are some of the causes of hypercalcemia. Stones may also form if the volume of urine is reduced, as occurs in dehydration, or if the acidity alters, as when the urine becomes infected.

Stones are a worldwide problem, although their incidence is higher in India and south-eastern Asia than in the Western world. Males are affected more frequently than females, and although some

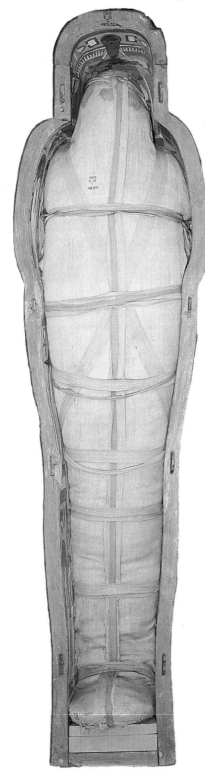

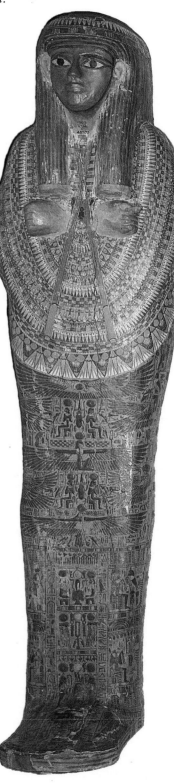

*The mummy and case of an
unnamed priestess from Thebes dates
back to 1050 B.C. When examined by
modern scientists, similar specimens
were found to contain renal stones—
a problem as old as humankind.*

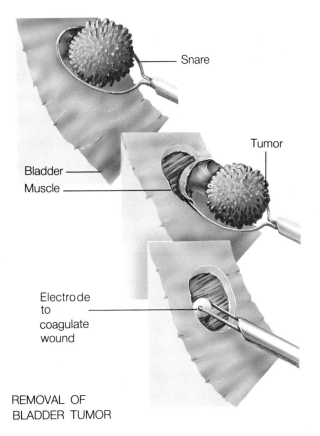

REMOVAL OF
BLADDER TUMOR

patients only have one stone, in fifty per cent of cases they are recurrent. An increase in renal stones has been associated with a sedentary lifestyle and living in a tropical climate with intermittent periods of dehydration.

The effect of a stone depends on its size. Very small stones (up to one-twelfth of an inch across) easily pass through the urinary tract without producing symptoms. Larger stones measuring more than one-third of an inch are retained in the renal pelvis, where they may increase in size but rarely produce symptoms. They may assume the shape of the pelvis, when they are called "staghorn" calculi. It is the stones that enter the ureter and then become stuck which give rise to renal colic. The pain may be a constant backache or a severe colicky pain which makes the patient roll around seeking relief. As the stone passes down the ureter, the pain often moves from the back or loin to the groin.

If a treatable cause can be identified, then appropriate measures can be taken. But in many cases a cause cannot be found, and these stones are called "idiopathic". Simple measures help to reduce recurrences, and the most valuable of these is to maintain a high fluid intake. This means four or six pints a day, which is difficult to achieve consistently—especially because most of the fluid should be water and because large amounts of tea, coffee and juices should therefore be avoided. Diets limiting calcium-rich foods (and thus severely restricting milk and milk products) have been tried. No definite evidence has been found to support claims for such diets, and indeed they may interfere with bone formation.

When simple measures fail, drug treatment can be tried; the drugs most commonly used are the thiazide diuretics. These reduce the amount of calcium which passes through the kidneys into the urine, but must be continued for months for any benefit to be achieved. If a stone is obstructing the kidney and does not move within a few days, crushing (litholapaxy) by ultrasound or surgical removal is indicated before any kidney damage occurs. In the past this involved major abdominal surgery, but great advances have now been made. By introducing an instrument through the urethra and bladder and into the ureter, a small gripping device called a Dormier basket can be used to trap the stone and remove it. It is sometimes difficult to perform successfully, and other techniques have also been developed. Stones can be removed by passing a tube from the abdominal wall to the kidney, forming a track called a nephrostomy, and this method provides easy access under local anesthetic. Recently a technique using shock waves delivered to a patient lying in a bath of water has been used to disrupt stones. It does not involve any surgery at all, and the particles from the stones are passed out in the urine.

Stones may form in the bladder for the same reasons as renal stones—especially if infection or a degree of obstruction is present — but they rarely cause problems.

High Blood Pressure

Because the kidneys play an essential role in the control of blood pressure, it is logical to expect that malfunction of the kidneys is related to hypertension, or high blood pressure. Indeed, hypertension can lead to renal disease and, conversely, kidney disorders may cause hypertension.

High blood pressure is one of the major causes of illness and eventual death in the Western world, and a significant cause of chronic renal failure. In ninety-five per cent of sufferers, the cause cannot be determined, and they are said to have essential hypertension. Diet has been implicated, and the role of salt intake is a particularly controversial subject. The Yanomamo Indians of South America are ideal examples of people who have extremely low levels of salt consumption; in them essential hypertension is rare. The amount of sodium in the body regulates blood volume and therefore blood pressure, and the kidneys are responsible for matching salt excretion to the amount eaten, to maintain a constant level in the body. Mild hypertension has been effectively controlled in some, but not all sufferers, by reducing salt intake.

Other dietary factors also seem to be important. Blood pressure falls slightly when people switch from normal to vegetarian diets, and the obese are considerably more at risk from hypertension than persons of average weight. One risk factor undisputed by nearly all physicians is the danger inherent in smoking tobacco, and a recently completed study concluded that giving up smoking is potentially more beneficial than drug therapy in reducing the mortality from mild hypertension.

Hypertension may be secondary to various disorders, especially those affecting the kidneys. They include disorders of the endocrine system, hormone-secreting tumors, renal tumors, narrowing (stenosis) of the renal arteries, stricture (coarctation) of the aorta, various forms of renal disease, polycythemia (an overall increase in red cell mass in the body), and treatment with some drugs (including oral contraceptives). The common denominator for many of these illnesses is an alteration of normal renal function, either directly or indirectly by some hormonal mechanism.

Narrowing, or stenosis, of the renal arteries results in an increase in the production of the hormone renin from the cells of the kidney. This was first shown experimentally by the American physiologist Harry Goldblatt, and the increase in blood pressure caused by renal artery stenosis is frequently referred to as Goldblatt hypertension. Patients suffering from glomerulonephritis or pyelonephritis also have hypertension caused by an overproduction of renin. Certain tumors themselves produce renin, upsetting the delicate balance of this hormone in the bloodstream and thus causing hypertension.

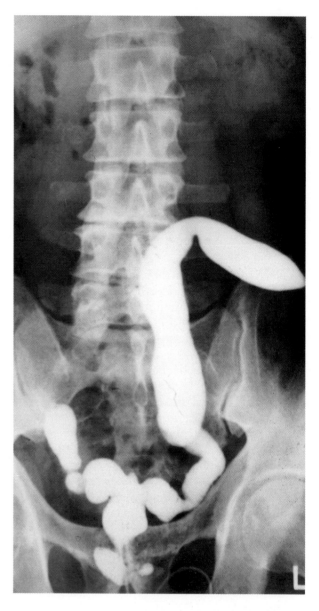

Tuberculosis of the renal tract is revealed in a retrograde pyelogram, in which the greatly swollen ureters are made to show up by injecting them with a radiopaque fluid through a catheter inserted via the bladder. The disorder is caused by bacteria and responds to long-term drug treatment.

*Stalactites in caves in the Blue Ridge
Mountains formed as water
percolating through limestone
evaporated, leaving calcium salts.
Excess calcium in the body can
accumulate as renal stones.*

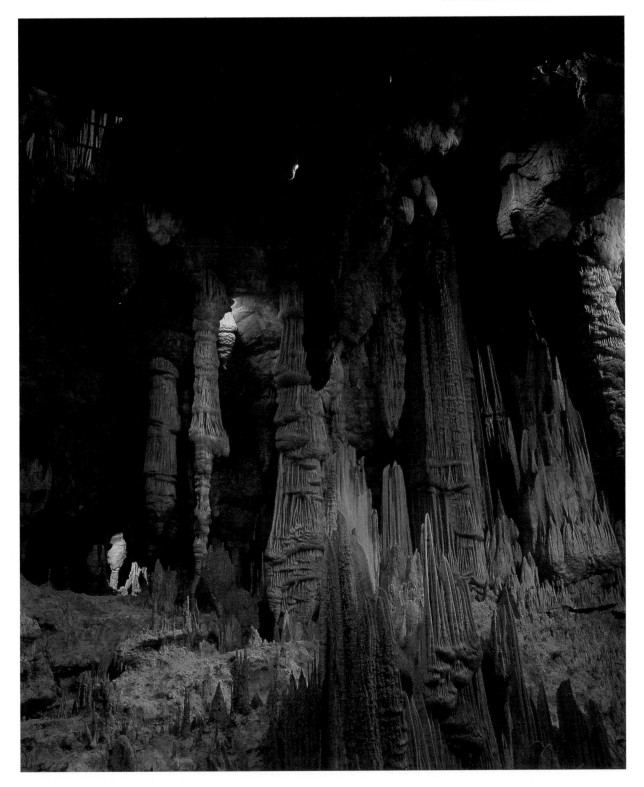

A staghorn calculus shows as the white spot near the center of this X ray of the kidney (left); the photograph (right) shows the stone after surgical removal. Renal stones may obstuct the flow of urine.

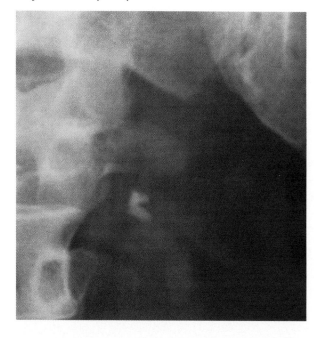
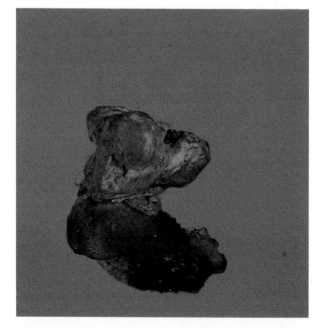

Other disorders of hormone production cause hypertension by an effect on the kidney. In the illness known as Conn's syndrome, named for the American internist, Jerome Conn, hypertension is caused by a decrease in sodium excretion brought about by overproduction of the hormone aldosterone, usually from a tumor of the adrenal glands. This condition is more common in women than in men, but less than one per cent of patients with hypertension have the disease. Excess production of the hormone hydrocortisone or cortisol (also by the adrenal glands) in Cushing's syndrome causes hypertension in a similar manner. Another hormonal cause is pheochromocytoma, in which a tumor in the adrenal gland or elsewhere secretes epinephrine. The symptoms resemble a state of fear, leaving the patient pale and sweating during an attack. Removal of the tumor brings about a complete recovery.

There is an increased incidence of hypertension among women taking the contraceptive pill. The risk is small, but blood pressure should be checked at regular intervals in all women taking the pill. The cause of the increase in blood pressure is thought to be associated with an activation of the renin-angiotensin system, and changes in the vessels within the kidney have been observed. Hyperten-

sion may also occur in pregnant women, when it may cause serious complications and jeopardize the health of the fetus. Women who were already hypertensive before pregnancy are particularly vulnerable. The cause of this type of hypertension is unknown, but salt and water retention, and hypersensitivity to the normal blood-pressure elevating hormones, are all thought to be involved.

In fewer than one per cent of hypertensives, malignant hypertension occurs, in which blood pressure rapidly and suddenly increases. Clinically it is diagnosed when the diastolic blood pressure is in excess of 130 millimeters of mercury, and is more common in young males, particularly blacks. Extensive damage to the kidneys occurs, commonly accompanied by proteinuria, and raised concentrations of urea and creatinine in the blood. The kidney damage leads, in turn, to increased renin production and worsening of the hypertension. Untreated, it leads to death within two years in ninety per cent of cases, and complications such as drowsiness, blindness and convulsions may occur if treatment is not started immediately.

Whatever the cause, hypertension, if untreated, leads to a deterioration of renal function, causing damage to the vessels within the kidney and leading to chronic renal failure. Therapy is aimed at

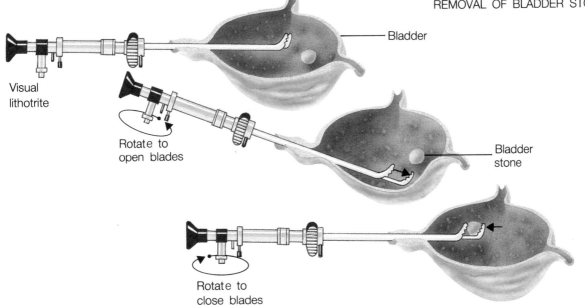

Considerable advancements have been made in the removal of bladder stones, including shattering them with sonic probes. An earlier technique called lithotrity, shown here, involves crushing the stone.

REMOVAL OF BLADDER STONE

Bladder

Visual
lithotrite

Rotate to
open blades

Bladder
stone

Rotate to
close blades

good control of blood pressure, after excluding or treating secondary causes of hypertension. If the blood pressure is reduced, the risk of death through renal failure, cerebrovascular accidents (strokes) and heart attacks can be lessened. In some patients a reduction in weight or a lower sodium intake may be sufficient to normalize blood pressure, whereas others require long-term drug therapy.

The volume of circulating blood is reduced by diuretic drugs, which increase the amount of water and sodium excreted by the kidneys. The drugs act directly on the cells of the kidney responsible for conserving water and reabsorbing sodium. Diuretics are frequently given with beta-blocking drugs, which inhibit the nerves serving the heart and blood vessels, so reducing the strength and speed of the heartbeat, and lowering the resistance to blood flow in peripheral blood vessels. Other drugs produce similar effects, but work by inhibiting the part of the central nervous system responsible for controlling blood pressure.

In recent years, two new groups of drugs have been introduced to treat hypertension. The calcium antagonists reduce the amount of calcium (necessary for contracting muscles) that enters the cells of the heart and blood vessels. This again lowers the peripheral resistance and reduces the force of the

heartbeat. The newest drugs are the ACE-inhibitors (ACE stands for angiotensin-converting enzyme), which work by blocking one of the important enzymes in the renin-angiotensin system, so reducing blood pressure.

Acute Renal Failure

In contrast to chronic renal failure, which may take months or even years to become serious, acute renal failure develops over hours or days. When the daily volume of urine produced is a pint or less, the condition is called oliguria, and at this stage waste products accumulate in the blood.

If the blood supply to the kidney is dramatically reduced because of bleeding — after an accident, for example — the kidneys fail temporarily but start working again if the blood loss is immediately made up. If the blood volume cannot be adequately replenished to increase blood pressure and restore the renal blood supply, then the kidney tubules start to die. Acute renal failure may be caused by direct damage to the kidney, such as severe glomerulonephritis or ingestion of a poison (such as antifreeze or carbon tetrachloride).

Sudden and complete obstruction of the urine flow may also cause acute renal failure. But these causes are potentially reversible, although recovery may take weeks. The amount of urea, creatinine and acid in the blood can rise dramatically. Potassium levels also increase, which interferes with the normal heartbeat, so cardiac arrest may result. Short-term dialysis may be required to tide the patient over a critical time, and a patient who is often too ill to eat must be nourished by intravenous feeding. It may be up to six weeks before the kidneys start producing urine again. The kidneys then enter a diuretic phase, when more urine is produced than normal, and the concentration of waste products slowly falls. It may be months or years before kidney function returns to normal, and in many patients recovery is never totally complete.

Chronic Renal Failure

The major cause of death from renal disease, chronic renal failure develops over a period of months or even years. Rarely, correction of the underlying disorder may result in a full recovery, but in most cases the progress of the disorder is unrelenting. The symptoms of chronic renal failure result from a build-up of metabolic waste products in the bloodstream, combined with a breakdown of the barriers that prevent leakage of substances from the blood into the urine, and a failure of other essential processes controlled by the kidneys.

Analysis of urine samples tells the clinician to what extent the normal barriers between blood and urine have collapsed, although the appearance of protein, red and white blood cells, and casts (prot-einaceous material precipitated into the tubules and washed down into the bladder) in the urine. Kidney function is assessed clinically by measuring the rate of excretion, or clearance, of the compound creatinine (a natural breakdown product of the body). Creatinine clearance approximates to the rate at which the kidneys filter fluid from the bloodstream (the glomerular filtration rate, or GFR), and is normally about one-quarter of a pint per minute.

Renal disease causes a' progressive fall in creatinine clearance. Only when it is reduced by more than sixty per cent do symptoms of renal illness start to appear, although the smaller reserve capacity means that traumatic events, such as surgery or gastrointestinal hemorrhage, may precipitate an episode of acute renal failure. This

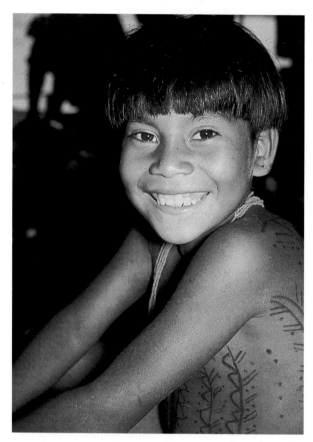

condition is sometimes referred to as "acute on chronic" renal failure.

As kidney failure progresses, symptoms of renal impairment begin to appear. When GFR is reduced to some twenty to thirty per cent of its normal value, the levels of various substances in the blood start to rise as their excretion by the kidneys falls below the rate of their formation. In particular, creatinine levels and the amount of blood urea nitrogen (BUN) increase. The amount of urine produced may also increase, as the concentrating power of the kidneys declines. If urine production exceeds six pints a day, the patient has polyuria — a need for frequent urination. Nocturia may also occur, in which the patient wakes frequently in the night to void urine. At this stage other symptoms such as hypertension and anemia become apparent as the kidneys lose their ability to function properly.

Anemia results because of a failure of the

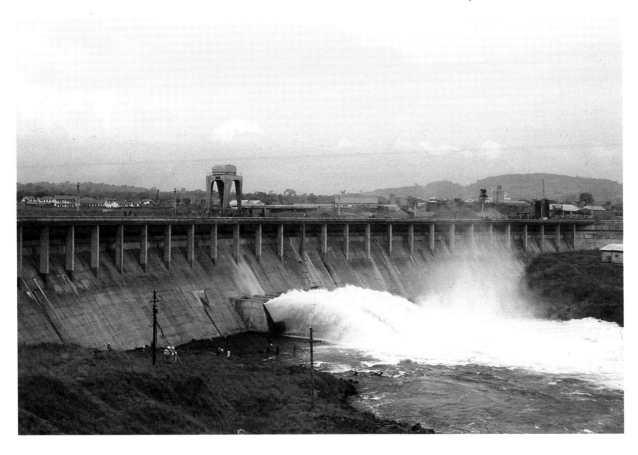

The regulation of the flow of water through a dam and the consequences of excessive flow are analogous to the control of blood pressure in the body. Excessive blood pressure can cause renal failure.

diseased kidney to produce erythropoietin, the hormone responsible for stimulating the production of red blood cells. As renal impairment increases, the production of the hormone falls, and so the number of red cells in the circulation declines. This is compounded by chronic blood loss, breakdown of red blood cells, and bone marrow suppression caused by the build-up of toxic substances in the bloodstream. The blood cells are often deformed, and are known as "burr" cells.

The increase in blood pressure is caused in part by derangement of the renin-angiotensin system and salt and water retention. It must be treated promptly, because high blood pressure accelerates the decline of the failing kidney. As GFR falls below twenty per cent of normal, the patient begins to display the classical symptoms of chronic renal failure. The production of urine declines (oliguria), or stops altogether (anuria), as the number of functional nephrons in the kidney decreases.

Patients feel lethargic and lose their appetites; nausea and vomiting are common, edema develops and, as the impairment becomes greater and greater, mental deterioration, confusion, and coma ensue. Many of the symptoms are thought to be caused by the build-up of metabolites of DNA and fragments of protein.

The blood becomes more acid than normal in renal failure because of the inability of the kidneys to excrete hydrogen ions. Other metabolic processes deranged by kidney failure include bone formation, which is dependent on the amount of calcium in the blood. Calcium levels fall, partly because of poor absorption of calcium from the diet, and partly because blood phosphate levels increase as renal excretion falls, which affects the normal balance between circulating calcium and calcium stores in bone. Calcium absorption is dependent on a metabolite of vitamin D produced by the kidney, and the level of this substance falls in renal failure.

SOURCES OF PROTEIN
IN THE URINE

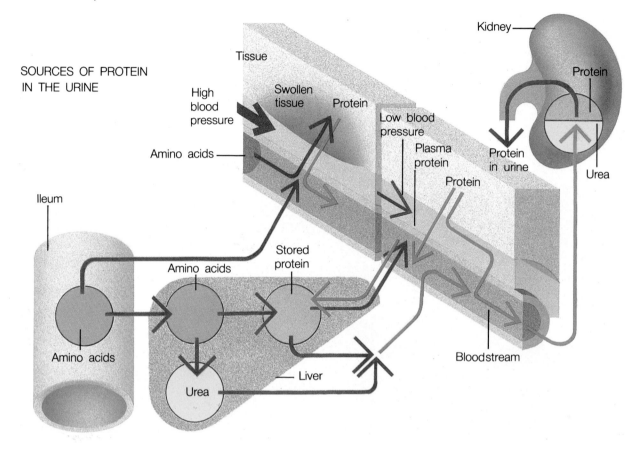

The decline in the level of calcium in the blood also stimulates the production of parathyroid hormone (PTH) from the parathyroid glands, and hyperparathyroidism results. In affected children bone growth is retarded and spontaneous fractures may occur. Vitamin D supplements and a reduction of dietary phosphate help to maintain blood calcium levels.

The treatment of chronic renal failure is aimed at reducing the symptoms, preventing complications such as congestive heart failure, and controlling problems such as vomiting and gastrointestinal bleeding. Primary causes such as obstruction and infections, which increase blood urea and so worsen the symptoms, must first be dealt with. Any hypertension must also be treated because of its contribution to renal failure. Other therapy is aimed at controlling salt and water intake, to reduce the load on the defective kidneys, and to prevent secondary complications. Urine output needs to be maintained at as high a level as possible to eliminate urea and toxic metabolites without precipitating heart failure, so that fluid intake has to be matched to the patient's ability to form urine. Protein intake is also reduced to help keep down the level of urea in the blood, relieving the patient of some of the symptoms of renal failure such as nausea and vomiting, although it does nothing to slow the course of the disease. The intake of protein has to be enough to replace losses in the urine. (A person weighing 125 pounds needs about an ounce of protein.) Proteins with high "biological value," such as those in eggs, milk and lean meat, help increase the utilization of urea, thereby reducing its level in the blood. A high-calorie diet is also essential to suppress the breakdown of protein in the patient's body.

By careful management during the progression of chronic renal failure, the quality of the patient's life can be maintained for some considerable time.

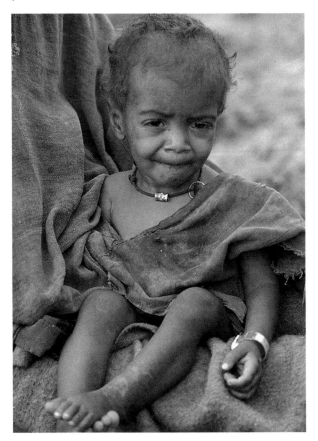

An Ethiopian famine victim shows some of the symptoms of a poor diet — including retarded bone growth, because of calcium deficiency which can, in turn, result from kidney failure.

Eventually, however, kidney function deteriorates to such a level that regular dialysis or renal transplantation is necessary.

The Prostate Gland

Located around the base of the bladder in men, the prostate gland produces secretions which are added to the semen. Only with increasing age do most men ever become aware of this gland, for at any time from their fifties it can gradually enlarge and start to obstruct the flow of urine. This happens because the central "hole" in the middle of the doughnut-shaped gland forms part of the urethra carrying urine from the bladder, and as the bulk of the prostate increases and becomes more rigid, the hole (or lumen) becomes smaller and the urethra is squeezed. As a result, the flow of urine becomes slower; it is also more difficult for the man to control the start and end of the stream, and to completely empty his bladder.

Often the first symptom elderly men notice is that they have to get out of bed several times a night to pass urine. This is a common problem, and more than eighty per cent of men over the age of eighty years have some degree of "prostatism." Fortunately the condition is easily recognized and treated, although repeat surgery is very occasionally required. It does, however, necessitate a major operation: a blood transfusion may be required. A fiber-optic instrument known as a resectoscope is passed along the urethra in the penis, and the narrowed lumen of the prostate is carefully cut wider using high-frequency electric current which simultaneously cauterizes.

When the urethra becomes completely blocked (usually in elderly men), "retention" occurs. It becomes almost impossible to pass urine, and pressure builds up as the bladder becomes more and more swollen. The pressure may damage the kidneys themselves, and retention usually necessitates an emergency admission to the hospital, where a catheter can be inserted to allow the bladder to empty. The blockage is then cleared in the way described, and once again all is well. The catheter is connected to a bag, allowing the patient to be fully mobile, and may be left in place for a few days or even weeks.

The lumen tissue removed when the prostate is resected is examined carefully under a microscope to see if there is any sign of cancer. Prostate cancers may be small enough to escape detection, causing no symptoms and not being evident as a lump. At this stage they are referred to as latent tumors, and no treatment is required. Most elderly men have such tumors which are discovered only by chance. Both the incidence and the effects seem to differ slightly between ethnic groups. Sometimes cancer of the prostate may spread in the same way as other cancers, and affect other organs in the body. Only lung cancer is more common in men, and prostate cancer is the third most common cause of death from cancer.

When such a cancer affects the prostate, an experienced physician can feel a hard lump, instead of a soft enlarged gland. The tumor may spread into the urethra and the bladder, or it may be carried through the blood vessels and lymphatic system into lymph nodes deep in the abdomen, or further

Prostate

Bladder

Prostate | Bladder

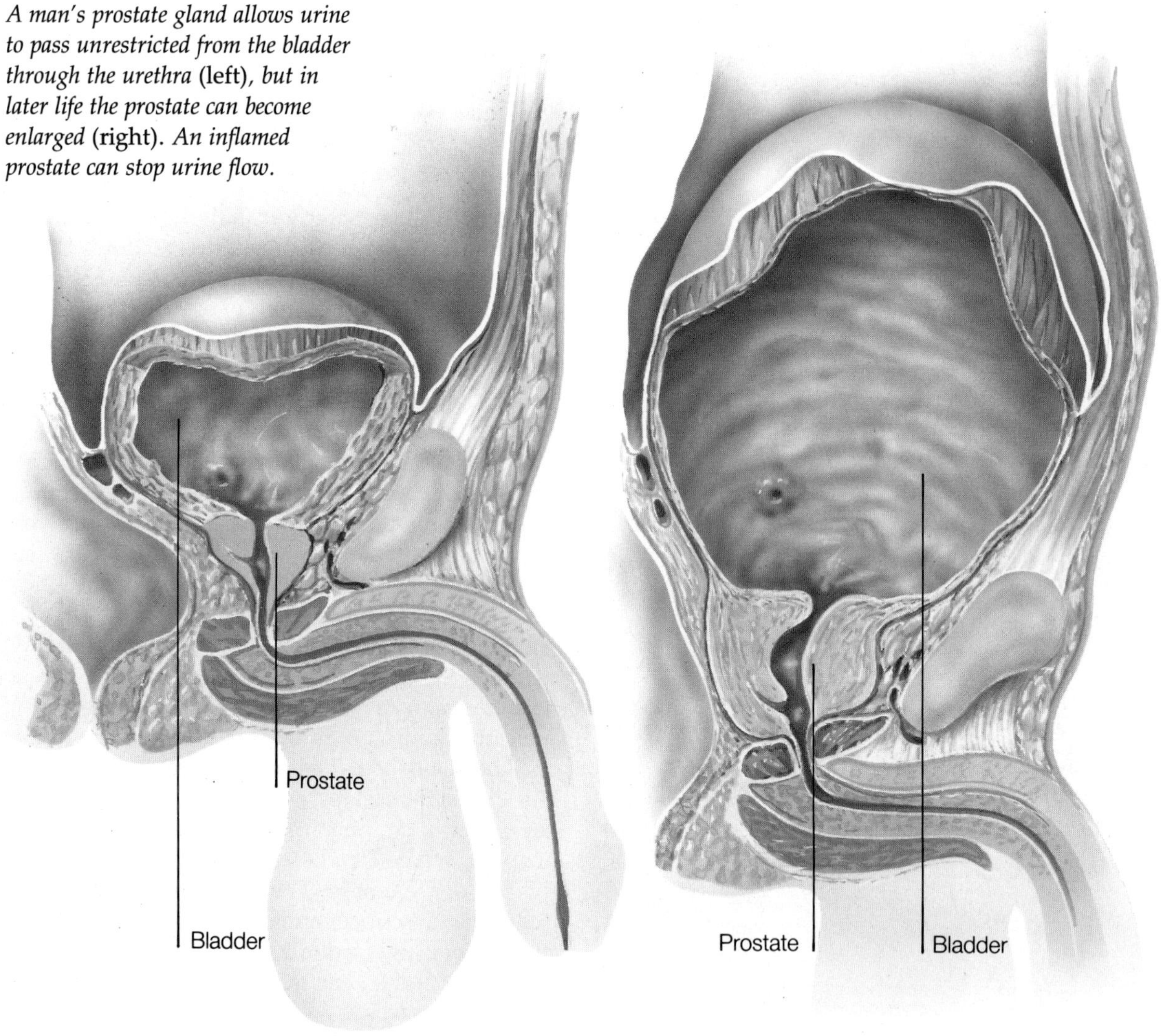

afield, especially into bone. One-third of patients thus affected survive for more than five years.

The male hormone testosterone is thought to play a part in the growth of such cancers, and so surgical removal of the testes is often employed to limit the disease. The spread of the disease and associated bone pain may be dramatically curtailed, but survival rates are unchanged. Instead of removing the testes, as commonly the effects of the male hormone are countered by giving estrogen, a female sex hormone. Many patients have been treated with the drug stilbestrol, which is chemically related to estrogen, but a side effect of such therapy is enlargement of the breasts. The chances of suffering hypertension, thrombosis and heart failure are also increased.

Tumors of the Urinary Tract

Different sites of the urinary tract are associated with tumors that vary, in both appearance and behavior. More than eighty per cent of tumors of the kidney itself are adenocarcinomas that frequently occur in middle-aged persons, affecting more men than women. Sometimes the patient notices a lump, or blood in the urine, but in other cases there is merely a mild fever. The kidney must be removed, but even so, fewer than one-half of such patients survive for five years after the diagnosis is made. The tumor may spread to the lungs, causing large, round secondary growths.

In children, a different type of kidney tumor occurs. Called a Wilm's tumor, the type represents one-third of all cancers in children; one-half of the children are under four years old. Their outlook has improved dramatically through treatment which combines surgery, radiotherapy and chemotherapy, so that ninety per cent are now alive five years after first diagnosis.

Cancer of the bladder accounts for three per cent of all deaths caused by cancer, and the number of

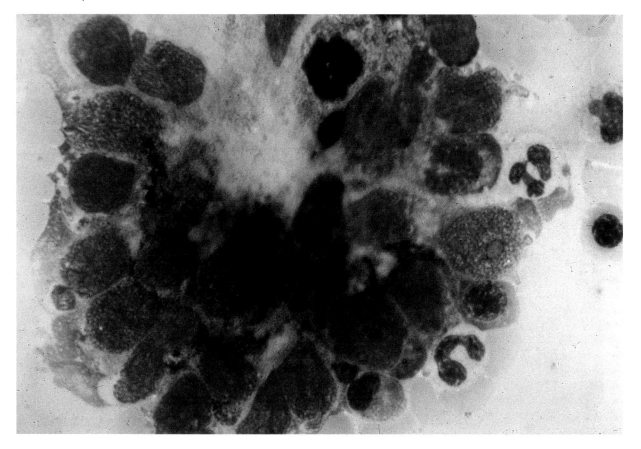

cases has been increasing over the last thirty years so that there are now 38,000 new cases of bladder cancer per year in the United States. Men are three times more likely to contract it than are women, largely because many cases are related to industrial exposure to carcinogens.

In 1894, the German surgeon Ludwig Rehn first noticed the development of cancers in aniline dye workers. Amines such as naphthylamine and benzidine, used in textiles, printing and plastics have been clearly associated with such cancers, and the incidence is three to four times higher in smokers than in nonsmokers. Alcohol and artificial sweeteners have caused tumors in experimental animals, but there is no definite proof of any such effect on humans. Similarly there is no evidence that people who live near chemical factories or use the products are at risk. The tumors grow from the skinlike lining of the bladder and ureters, and most are of the type known as transitional cell car-

cinomas. They may grow to form frondlike masses in the bladder, and with time spread through the wall. Usually they can be controlled by excising the tumor using a cystoscope (an endoscope for looking inside the bladder), but sometimes the whole bladder may have to be removed.

Inability to Control Urination

Incontinence, the inability to control the passing of urine, is a very common problem in the elderly, often because of senile dementia, stroke or merely increasing confusion. In these people the nerves to the bladder still function normally, but the voluntary control is lost. Even in elderly people who are not incontinent, there is a loss of the warning period between filling of the bladder and reflex emptying, and so they notice increasing frequency and urgency. This can usually be kept within manageable limits, but a short illness — such as a chest infection — may result in a loss of control and a period of incontinence. Careful nursing care is required so that the skin does not ulcerate, and the use of plastic panties, pads or rubber appliances may be indicated.

When control is completely lost — and especially if the patient is bedridden — a catheter may be the most suitable way to manage incontinence. A catheter is a soft rubber tube, which is inserted into the bladder and connected to a plastic bag. Urinary tract infections are common when a catheter is in place — which may be for several weeks or months at a time — and so thorough hygiene must be employed to prevent them.

In elderly men, a large prostate gland or other obstruction can block the urinary flow and incontinence results from "overflow." In elderly women, prolapse of the uterus may be associated with incontinence. Infection can result in incontinence in any age group.

Stress incontinence often affects younger women, especially after childbirth. The muscles of the pelvic floor become weak and the sphincter at the bottom of the bladder lax, so that if the woman laughs, coughs or sneezes, the resulting increase in intra-abdominal pressure allows a small volume of urine to leak. This may be only an occasional problem — which is merely a nuisance — although more severe problems may have to be treated by means of surgery.

The nerves to the bladder may be damaged by disorders such as multiple sclerosis, diabetes or by trauma — for example following a car crash. The result varies according to the site of the nerve damage, but recurrent and severe infections are common. The bladder may contract frequently without emptying completely, or it may distend and just overflow, like a sink with the plug in and the tap left running. In paraplegics, self-catheterization several times a day sometimes works well, but in many patients a long-term catheter is the only solution.

Bed-wetting (enuresis) may occur in completely normal children, who may not be reliably dry at night until the age of eight or nine years. Some may have infections which make them more likely to wet the bed. When there is no reason to suspect emotional problems it is important to be sympathetic but firm with such children, and ensure that

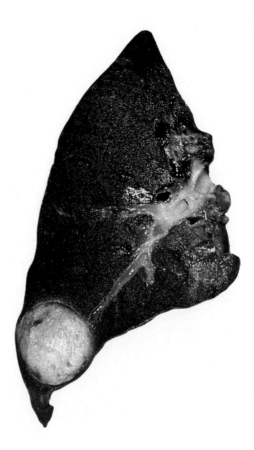

Wilm's kidney tumor occurs in children, and can be treated by surgery and with drugs. Occasionally it spreads to the lungs (as shown here), causing a large secondary growth.

they use the toilet frequently and regularly during the day. Practice in holding urine and stopping nighttime drinks may help; some medications are available which increase nighttime control.

The Causes of Gout

Gout has been familiar to physicians for centuries, and was first described by Hippocrates in 460 B.C. Galen attributed gout to debauchery, intemperance and a hereditary trait. The caricature of a well-to-do, port-drinking male gout sufferer is well known, but not all sufferers are fat, elderly men, and not all cases are caused by drinking port. Gout is, however, extremely rare in children and in women of childbearing age.

The classic pattern of gout is swollen joints of the toes and fingers, which become extremely painful. Sometimes only one joint, usually the big toe, is affected. The symptoms are caused by the crystallization of uric acid in the joint, causing swelling,

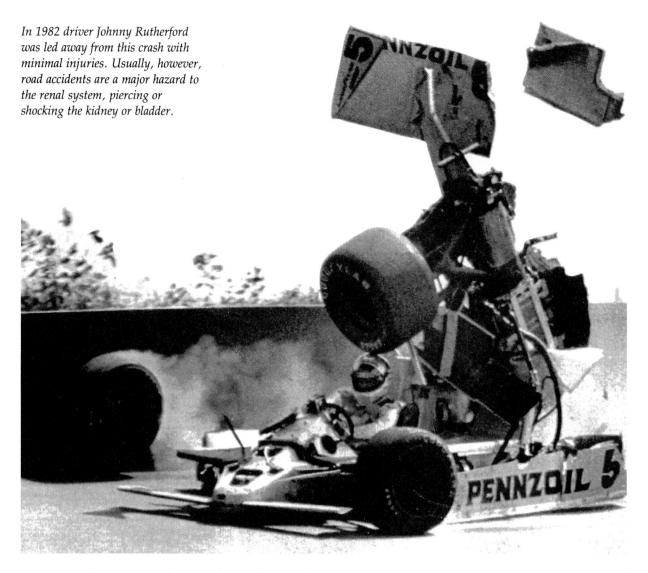

In 1982 driver Johnny Rutherford was led away from this crash with minimal injuries. Usually, however, road accidents are a major hazard to the renal system, piercing or shocking the kidney or bladder.

redness and severe pain. Frequently a sufferer with gout in the toes cannot wear shoes. When the disease has been present for some years, small nodules called gouty tophi may develop, often on the edge of the ear, which can also be painful. Precipitation of urates in the kidney, by damaging the tubules, may cause renal failure.

Gout is caused by an increase in the level of uric acid in the blood (hyperuricemia). Uric acid is a normal metabolic breakdown product of purines, which are some of the building blocks for DNA. In most cases the reason for the increase in uric acid cannot be found. The kidneys normally excrete it, but can cope with only a small amount at a time. If the concentration of uric acid in the urine increases, urate stones may form. There are also rare hereditary conditions which give rise to gout, and many cases run in families. It may also be caused by drugs, such as those used to treat leukemia. When leukemia is treated in this way, many leukemic cells die at the same time, releasing a massive amount of urate which can block renal tubules and cause acute renal failure.

Diet also plays a role in gout. Rich foods — particularly a lot of meat, which has a high purine content — and alcohol, which interferes with uric acid excretion, contribute to the illness. There are, however, other factors, such as the genetic makeup of the individual, which allow gout to develop. Preventive measures are frequently successful. They include a diet containing less meat, reduced alcohol consumption, and a high fluid intake. The drug allopurinol, which prevents the formation of uric acid, is useful in severe cases.

Systemic Diseases and the Kidney

Any systemic disease — one that has an effect on the whole body — can damage the kidneys, but those that affect the blood vessels are particularly implicated. Systemic lupus erythematosus (SLE),

David M. Hume

The Triumph of Transplantation

Described after his tragic and untimely death as "brash but immensely likable," "belligerently good-natured," and "cheeky, occasionally argumentative, but sadly missed," David Milford Hume was evidently a rather forceful character in the world of renal surgery specialists. Always at the forefront of knowledge in his field, he applied that same dynamism to his medical research.

Hume was born in 1917, and grew up always wanting to do medical research. Gaining his doctorate at the University of Chicago in 1943, he joined the staff of the Peter Bent Brigham Hospital in Boston, and remained there until 1951. Then, at the relatively early age of thirty-four, he became Director of the Laboratory for Surgical Research at Harvard Medical School, a post he retained until 1956, although within that period his work in kidney transplants was interrupted by a second tour of duty in the US Navy in the Korean War. Thereafter, until his death, he was Professor of Surgery and Chairman of the Department at the Medical College of Virginia.

For many years, beginning at the time they were together at the Peter Bent Brigham Hospital, Hume and John P. Merrill were the leading

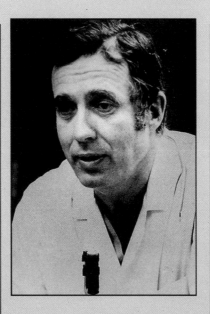

specialists in the world at renal surgery. Together they pioneered kidney transplants at the hospital, and although Merrill—who remained at the hospital—concentrated on transplantation from then on, Hume—who moved on— turned rather to trying to find out how to make kidney grafts (from donor to patient) more successful. In both cases, the main problem was tissue rejection, a subject on which Hume and Merrill constantly conferred.

When Hume reached Virginia, he and Merrill continued to correspond. By around 1960, Merrill had developed new surgical techniques affecting the location of transplanted

kidneys; Hume in the meantime was experimenting with irradiation of patients as therapy to reduce tissue rejection. Two years later, a form of chemotherapy for the same purpose was added to other treatments, and the results were good enough for Hume to be able to claim that his methods of grafting and transplantation were "at last showing signs of coming of age."

By the later 1960s, anti-rejection drug therapy had been considerably refined. In all transplants the removal of both original kidneys of the patient had become standard procedure, and the success rate of Hume's transplants between relatives went up to over 60 per cent—but was still nowhere near as good with kidneys taken from cadavers or non-relatives.

At the same time, Hume had other interests. He was as deeply involved in surgical endocrinology—in fact he was responsible for the first quantitative bio-assay for serum adenocorticotropic hormone (ACTH). Regarded as brilliant in both of his fields, Hume was also well respected for his extremely thorough methods of analyzing results.

He died flying his plane from a medical visit to the West Coast in 1973.

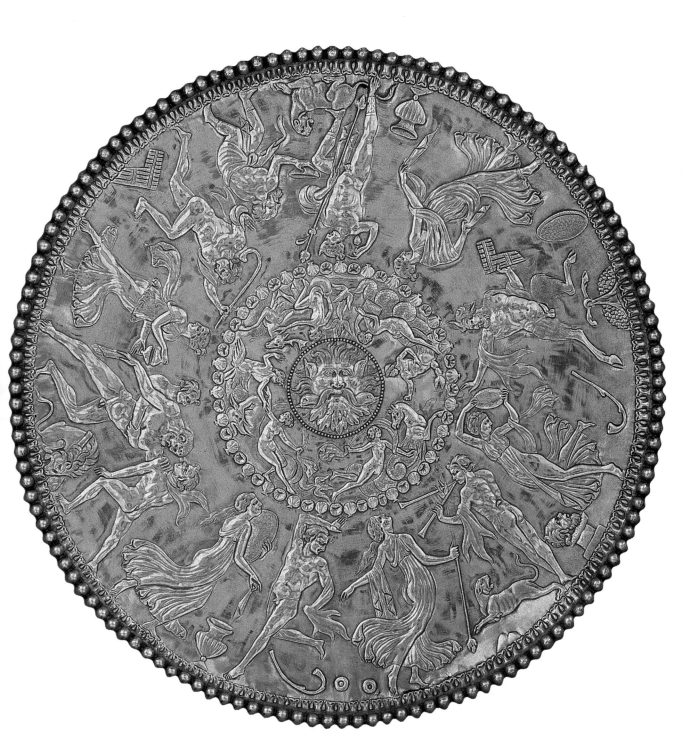

The Roman scholar Galen attributed
the cause of gout to loose living,
which is not peculiar to any one age.
Here the Great Dish, a piece of
Roman silver, depicts an orgy with a
drunken Hercules being supported
(left center).

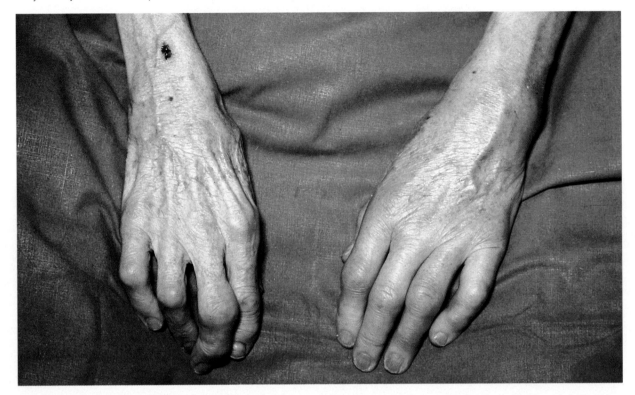

for example, is an inflammatory disease involving a wide variety of organs. It is nine times more prevalent in women than in men, and most cases occur during the childbearing years. It almost always causes some damage to the kidneys, and many forms of glomerulonephritis are associated with it. SLE may cause a characteristic skin rash across the bridge of the nose, joint pain, and inflammation of the heart, brain or lungs, as well as of the kidneys. Steroid drugs are usually prescribed to help suppress the inflammation.

Polyarteritis nodosa is a disorder that affects arteries throughout the body, causing weakening of the vessel walls and inflammation. Young men are more commonly affected than women, and many have previously been infected with hepatitis B virus. The effects may be devastating, the young patients suffering strokes and heart attacks. Many develop renal failure, although this may take many years to become apparent.

Renal injury is common in people suffering from diabetes mellitus, with damage to the glomeruli and the vessels serving them as a dominant feature.

The exact cause remains a mystery, but many scientists have studied the relationship between renal damage and the appearance of various carbohydrates around the glomerulus. The search for the cause is particularly intense because about one in every three diabetics with juvenile, or insulin-dependent, diabetes goes on to develop renal failure. The characteristic condition, with nodules of material in the glomeruli, was first described by the German-born American pathologist Paul Kimmelsteil and the British physician Clifford Wilson, and has been named the Kimmelsteil-Wilson syndrome. It generally appears between twelve and twenty-two years after the onset of diabetes, and heralds final renal failure some four to five years later. The patient then needs dialysis or a transplantation operation.

The renal arteries of diabetic patients also show advanced atherosclerosis. At any age diabetics are more likely to suffer from urinary tract infections, especially if the control of blood sugar is poor, because bacteria grow more profusely in sugary urine. Renal disease is more frequent, severe, and

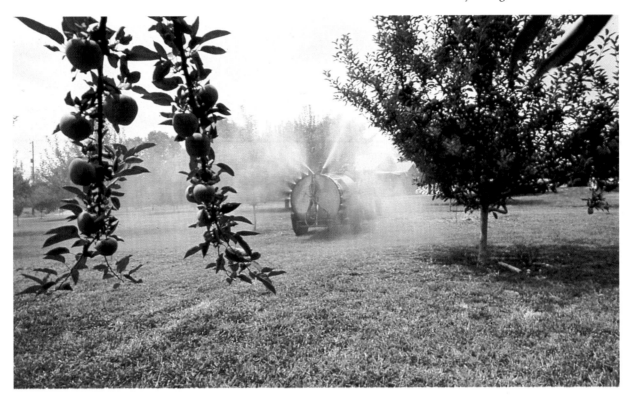

Many of the chemicals used for spraying crops to control pests are toxic. If they are accidently ingested, they pass to the kidneys, whose function it is to remove them, at the risk of damage.

progressive in insulin-dependent diabetes than in maturity-onset diabetes.

Amyloidosis is a curious disease in which an unusual protein, amyloid, fills up the blood vessels, not only in the kidney (which is almost invariably involved) but also in the heart, liver, spleen and many other organs. Sometimes amyloidosis accompanies a blood disease in which excessive immunoglobulin is produced; in other patients there may be a chronic inflammation, such as rheumatoid arthritis. In many cases, however, no cause can be determined. Once amyloid is found in the kidney, the outlook is poor and renal failure usually occurs within a year or two.

Henoch-Schönlein purpura, named after the German pediatrists Edouard Henoch and Johann Schönlein, is a disease that affects principally young children. Apart from having hematuria and proteinuria through renal damage, patients develop a characteristic rash over the buttocks and lower limbs, and have abdominal pains. The cause of the disease is still unknown, but it frequently follows throat or chest infections, and some immune mechanism defect is probably to blame. A progressive glomerulonephritis may develop, and a proportion of patients eventually develop chronic renal failure.

Drugs may also cause kidney damage, and such damage, or renal failure itself, necessitates caution in drug therapy because of increases in concentration and toxicity. A hypersensitivity reaction affecting blood vessels in the kidney can occur with antibiotics such as penicillin and sulfonamides. Gold and penicillamine, used in the treatment of rheumatoid arthritis, can cause a membranous glomerular nephritis, and the antihypertensive drug hydralazine may, rarely, induce a syndrome resembling systemic lupus erythematosus. Obstruction to the kidney caused by fibrous growth around the ureters (retroperitoneal fibrosis) may result from therapy with drugs such as ergotamine (a powerful alkaloid drug derived from ergot, sometimes used in the treatment of migraine). Accidental ingestion of poisons such as the weedkiller paraquat produces rapid renal failure and lung damage.

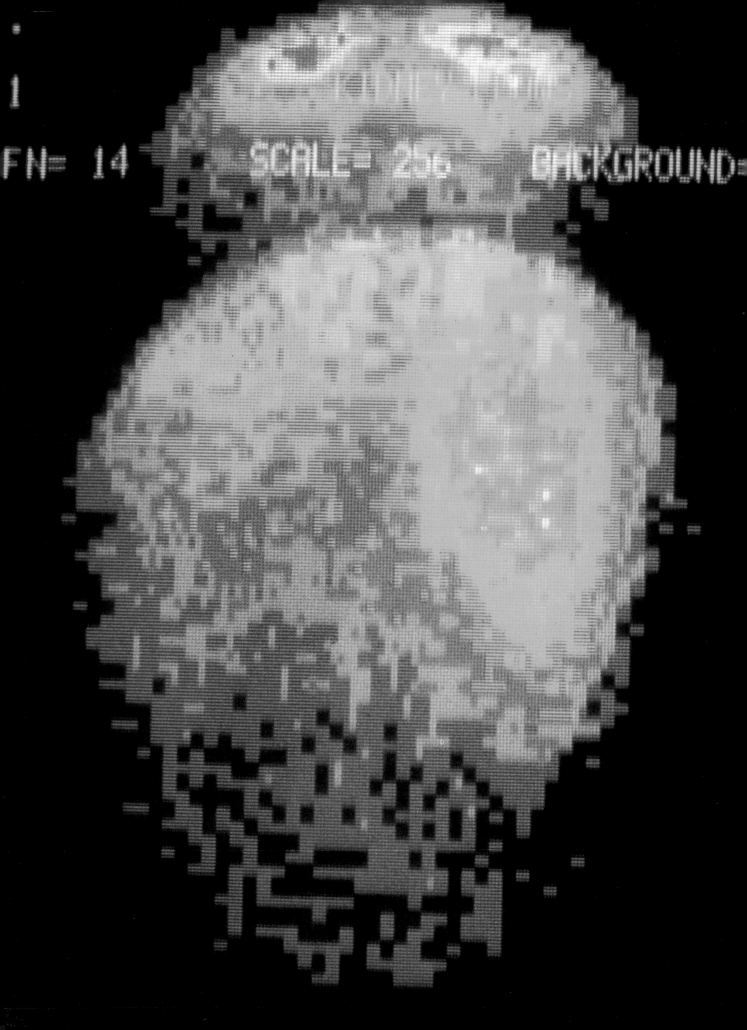

Chapter 5

Renal Replacement

The kidney was the first organ in the body whose chief function was duplicated by a machine, and the first to be successfully replaced by a donor organ. Today it is still by far the most commonly transplanted organ. Since the late 1940s, the methods developed for renal replacement therapy have helped to advance transplant programs for many other organs, such as the heart and lungs.

It is ironic that war often stimulates remarkable advances in medicine which subsequently offer to the peacetime civilian population the benefits of research that might not otherwise have been carried out. There are many examples: the treatment of burns for the aircrew of World War II offered new hope for burn victims everywhere; and the treatment of terrorist bomb victims has greatly enlarged the scope for treating those who suffer multiple injuries in road accidents. The kidney machine was developed to treat casualties in Europe during World War II.

During the intense bombing campaigns on major English cities in the early 1940s, people were often rescued from the rubble miraculously still alive, only to die of kidney failure a few days later because prolonged crushing by the rubble had produced poisonous toxins in the kidneys with which, even when function was restored, they were unable to cope. Similarly, wounded or burned soldiers could be saved by an immediate blood transfusion and yet go into renal failure and die some days after the initial trauma because shock (the massive loss of blood) had lowered their blood pressure to such an extent that the kidney tissue started to die. Replacing the blood with a transfusion was thus not enough; the kidneys were damaged beyond repair, urine production shut down completely and the patients died of acute kidney failure.

What was particularly frustrating to the surgeons at the time was that, although many patients died, there were others who suffered acute kidney failure for a few days but, once through it, recovered their

A computerized axial tomograph – a CAT scan – presents an X-ray image of a kidney in a chosen cross-section. New techniques such as this have greatly helped advance research into the kidney and its disorders.

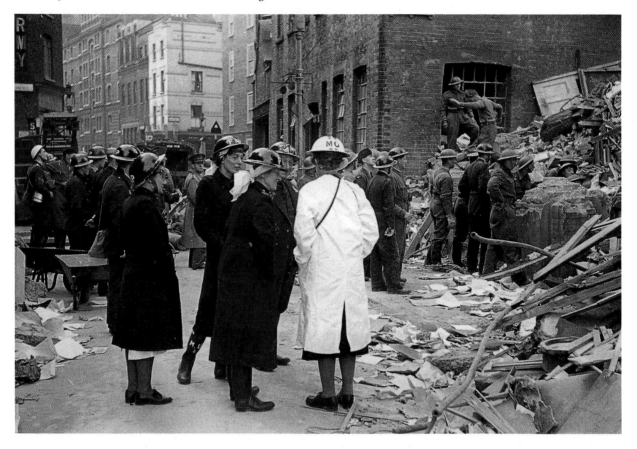

kidney function. This seemed to indicate that in many cases the kidneys were not permanently damaged. Some way had to be found to tide a patient over the period of renal failure so as potentially to achieve a full recovery from the devastating injuries.

The healthy kidney acts as a filter, separating waste products, salts and water from the other components of the blood. When the kidneys fail to produce urine, waste products such as urea (formed when proteins are broken down) accumulate in the blood. These waste materials are toxic, and when the levels eventually become high enough, the body is no longer able to survive and the victim dies. It usually takes between seven and fourteen days for toxins in the blood to reach fatal levels, but if the rate of the build-up of waste is reduced, survival may be prolonged.

Willem Kolff, a Dutch physician, developed a method of imitating the filtration function of the kidney. His achievement is the more remarkable because he developed his artificial kidney in the Netherlands during the wartime occupation by the Germans. Using only the most primitive resources, he manufactured the first effective kidney machine. News of Kolff's achievement reached Dr John Putnam Merrill, a physician with the American VIII Army after the Allied invasion of Europe. Merrill arranged for Kolff to emigrate to the United States, and together they developed an artificial kidney at Boston's Peter Bent Brigham Hospital.

Artificially Filtering Blood

All artificial kidneys work on the scientific principle of dialysis, the passage of small molecules from one fluid to another across a special membrane. The membrane is semipermeable: it has numerous small holes that allow small molecules to pass through but that keep out large molecules (such as proteins). If the semipermeable membrane is

William J. Kolff

Deviser of the Artificial Kidney

Dutch people tend to be both ingeniously practical and modestly determined to further the use of their creative ideas. Willem Johan Kolff—perfector of several types of dialysis machines ("artificial kidneys") and creator of various other machines, devices and techniques—is a supreme example. He began his work at a time when no regular renal dialysis of any kind was available to patients, since when—largely through his research—it has become possible for all patients with chronic or acute kidney complaints to be dialyzed, in a hospital or even at home.

Kolff was born in Leiden, Holland, in February 1911. Educated at the State University there, he received his doctorate in 1938. Just before the outbreak of World War II he transferred from the University's pathology department in Leiden to that in Groningen, where he built his first dialyzing apparatus and began work on refinements to improve it. This lasted only until 1941, however, when the effects of the invasion of the Netherlands by the Germans obliged him to take up a position as internist at a hospital in the old city of Kampen.

Conditions were difficult in Kampen, but Kolff persisted in

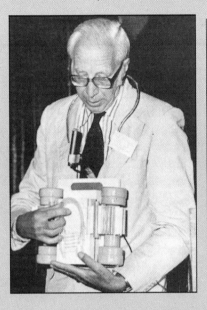

his research and was allocated a laboratory, equipment, and a staff of technicians; he also managed, despite the privations of the war, to get help from local manufacturers toward obtaining various bits of machinery for his dialyzers. Use of his device on a patient was inaugurated in March 1943 —the first external dialysis ever successfully carried out. But it was not for a few more years that the optimal dialyzing medium was established, and in the meantime results with the early patients were disappointing.

Following a trip to Boston, Mass., in 1947—where he donated the blueprints of his latest machine to Peter Bent Brigham Hospital, later to

become famous for kidney dialysis and research into transplantation—Kolff emigrated to the United States, and in 1950 became Professor of Clinical Investigation at the Cleveland Clinical Foundation. Eight years on he accepted the additional post of Head of the Department of Artificial Organs, and remained at Cleveland in both capacities until 1967.

At that time he took up a similarly senior combination of virtually identical posts at the College of Medicine at the University of Utah. And it was from there that he eventually retired.

Kolff's first invention was the rotating drum artificial kidney, in which twenty yards of cellophane tubing passed blood from one end of a revolving drum to the other, the lower half of the drum being immersed in dialyzing fluid.

Later dialyzers did not require the drum to rotate and were based on a notion of mobility and disposability. In Cleveland, Kolff used seven beer cans in his initial plan for the twin-coil artificial kidney now in use all over the world. Further examples of his ingenuity were experiments in dialysis using pressure cookers, washing machines and the nose-cone of a rocket.

The artificial kidney machine mimics the function of the damaged organ it has replaced by filtering potentially dangerous waste products from other components of the blood. The principle by which it does so is known as dialysis. Once the patient is connected to the machine, blood containing cells, proteins, salts and toxins is pumped to the dialyzer, where a semipermeable membrane (below right) allows waste products and unwanted salts to diffuse across into a solution of de-ionized water and dialysate concentrate, while blood cells and plasma proteins, which are too large to pass through, are left behind.

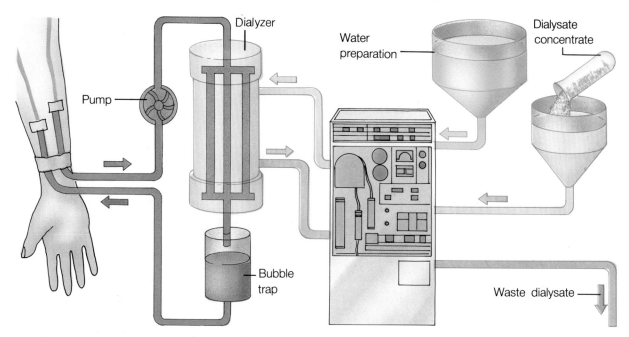

stretched between a fluid containing salt and protein on one side and pure water on the other, then the salt passes through the membrane until its concentration is the same on both sides, but all the proteins stay in the original fluid. If the initial salt and protein solution has a small volume and the water a large volume, then the salt concentration following dialysis is very low on both sides of the membrane because the salt has been diluted in the large volume of water. But the protein remains at the original concentration, because it is trapped in its original volume of fluid.

Kidney machines work on the same principle. Blood — containing cells, plasma proteins, salts and wastes — is on one side of the semipermeable membrane and a special salt solution, designed to contain the right mixture and concentration of small molecules, is on the other. Waste molecules and unwanted salts diffuse through the membrane into the salt bath and the blood cells and plasma proteins stay behind. Because the volume of fluid in the salt bath is large, the concentration of wastes is rapidly diluted so that the levels in the blood quickly become nearly normal.

Early kidney machines were intended for short-term use, generally for dialysis only once or a few times while a patient's damaged kidneys were given a chance to recover. Once it became possible to treat acute renal failure successfully, however, the prospect of using the same method to treat chronic renal failure became attractive. Could a patient with permanent kidney failure be kept alive through the use of an artificial kidney? Such chronic dialysis presented a whole series of technical and ethical problems, most of which were solved during the late 1950s and early 1960s. By the mid-1980s chronic dialysis has kept thousands of individuals alive for years.

The basic principle of dialysis is simple; the actual engineering required to connect a person to a machine, to pump blood safely through the device, and to return the blood to the patient is complex. Many precautions have to be taken in order to prevent catastrophic bleeding, the blood from clotting in the machine, the poisoning of the patient by the contents of the dialysis bath, or the introduction of infection into the system.

The process of connecting a person's blood vessels to the tubes of the artificial kidney is known as vascular access, and poses many problems for patients with renal failure. For one or two dialyses only, it is feasible to sacrifice a small artery and vein by connecting them directly onto the machine. Blood flows from the artery through the coiled

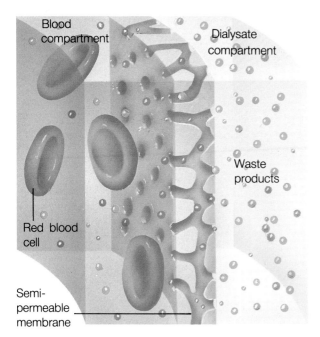

Blood compartment

Dialysate compartment

Red blood cell

Waste products

Semi-permeable membrane

membrane immersed in the dialysis bath, and then back through the vein. The reason this method can be employed only a few times is because the artery and the vein which are utilized become permanently damaged — and there are only few such vessels that can be spared.

One solution is to make a relatively long-term connection between an artery and a vein using a piece of silicone rubber tubing, called a Quinton-Shribner shunt for the doctors who invented it. A loop of the shunt is left outside the body so that the tubes of the dialysis machine can be connected to it through a joint. Eventually, however, the vessels supplying the shunt close off through clotting, and the shunt must be moved to a new site. Nevertheless, with a shunt the blood vessels involved last far longer; months, or even years, of dialysis can be accomplished through one site. The Quinton-Schribner shunt finally made long-term dialysis a practical possibility.

An alternative to the rubber shunt is a minor surgical operation to create what is known as a fistula, by which an artery and vein are surgically joined together. This lowers the risk of introducing infection because both vessels remain covered with a protective coating of skin; the risk of thrombosis (clotting) is also decreased. Once connected to an artery, the vein dilates because of the increase in blood flow and pressure, and thus forms an easy target for needles attached to the tubing of the dialysis machine.

Once the patient is connected to the machine a small amount of heparin — a drug that overrides the blood's tendency to clot — is added to the blood to prevent it forming clots in the tubes of the machine. In some patients the effects of the heparin have later to be reversed at the end of the dialysis run, usually by adding some of the protein protamine to the blood.

The composition of the fluid in the dialysis bath is crucial to both short- and long-term effects of dialysis. Either too little or too much salt may have catastrophic effects on the body's delicately balanced chemistry. Another constituent is a complex sugar, and how much is present affects the amount of water removed from the blood. If there is too much, the effects can be very similar to a serious hemorrhage. Too little, however, causes an accumulation of excess fluid in the body of the patient, which may spill over into the lungs and cause pulmonary edema.

Recently, longer-term problems have been uncovered relating to the composition of the water used to make up the dialysis fluid. In some areas the water ordinarily supplied has a high natural aluminum content. This is now known to be dangerous: a gradual increase in the aluminum levels in dialysis patients can have devastating effects, even to the extent of eventually producing neurological damage. Where aluminum toxicity is likely to prove a problem, deionized or distilled water has to be used to make up the dialysis bath.

Increasing Independence

When chronic hemodialysis first became practical, the process was carried out in the hospital. A patient was hospitalized, connected to a machine and dialyzed for ten to sixteen hours at a time. Usually necessary two or three times a week, the operation was clearly time-consuming and expensive. It was also available only in a limited number of large medical centers. People who lived in parts of the country where there was no such center were obliged to move house in order to receive the regular treatment without which they would die.

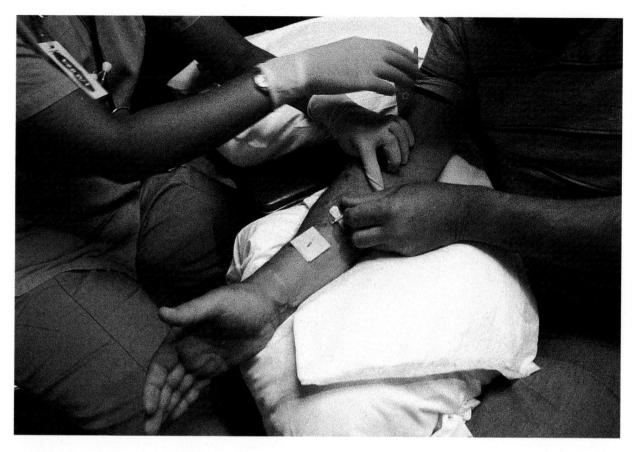

Family life could be completely disrupted by frequent visits to the hospital; vacations or extended business trips were impossible. Some — perhaps most — of these restrictions have now been partially overcome by technical advances.

Once all the procedures involved in setting up a dialyzer and attaching it to the patient's shunt or fistula were well understood and routinely practiced, it became clear that many patients were perfectly capable of dialyzing themselves. Gradually, many nurses and doctors found themselves relegated to an advisory role toward those patients who had a real desire — and were able — to do what they could for themselves. Such an attitude is doubly healthy because self-help not only restores a person's independence and physical mobility, but also helps those who may have come to feel overwhelmed by fate to assert themselves once again as in control of their own destiny.

Home dialysis has been greatly aided by the miracles of modern technology, resulting in simpler, more compact machines, prepackaged salt solutions, and "foolproof" connectors. But despite the technical wizardry involved, however, the critical factor remains the patient's motivation. To be suitable for a home dialysis program, an individual must be prepared and able to learn an exacting routine that must be followed with meticulous attention to every detail. A devoted relative or friend who lives in or nearby, and who can help with setting up and coming off the machine, is also essential. The patient must be psychologically assessed and deemed to have a stable personality and should enjoy at least one stable social relationship.

Home dialysis obviously causes a certain amount of disruption to home life. Usually, a small room in the home has to be reserved solely for the kidney machine and its accompanying paraphernalia. Having its own special location helps to maintain the vital sense of routine ritual involved (and means it does not have to be moved to be cleaned). Going on and coming off a dialyzer at home has a "check list" of procedure much like the one used by airplane pilots before take-off or landing. High technology, fastidious attention to detail, and a strong sense of self-preservation all combine for a successful program; home dialysis works well every day and can soon become part of a person's routine. For someone whose personality or surroundings are judged not to be ideal, however, hospital-based dialysis is still an invaluable option.

Another advance that has made dialysis patients more independent is the miniature portable

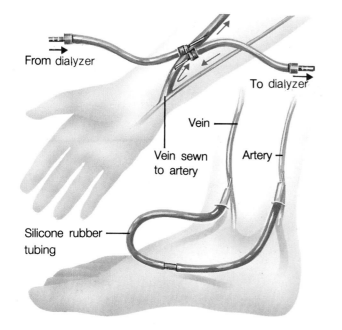

From dialyzer

To dialyzer

Vein

Vein sewn to artery

Artery

Silicone rubber tubing

kidney, a device that allows a patient to move away from the home or hospital installation for a short period. The miniature kidney is suitable only for a few runs, but it allows a patient to take a real vacation involving a wider degree of mobility and a stay of two or three weeks away from homebase. Now that regular hemodialysis is available to many thousands of people, there is a demand for vacation dialysis centers. These facilities cater for all kinds of vacationers, but also include a fully-staffed dialysis center for people who require it.

Further Developments

Hemodialysis is completely successful for many people. For others, though, it does present drawbacks — some physical, some emotional and some purely social — and for these people, alternative methods of removing body wastes and water from the body have been developed.

Instead of an artificial semipermeable membrane, for example, one of the body's own natural semipermeable membranes can be utilized. Such a membrane, which covers the abdominal wall cavity and wraps around the organs within it, is called the peritoneum, and has an enormous surface area because it covers all the folding contours of the intestines. It is certainly large enough for the

exchange of the small waste molecules. For peritoneal dialysis, fluid is run into the abdomen through a rubber tube (a catheter) and wastes are exchanged into the fluid through the peritoneum just as they are in an artificial kidney. The dialysis fluid is removed, and fresh fluid added, so that over a period of hours accumulated toxins and water are washed out from the blood.

Long-term peritoneal dialysis was made possible by the invention of a special flexible, non-irritating catheter first introduced in 1968 and called a Tenckhoff catheter for its developer. The tube is placed through the skin into the abdominal cavity and is intended to remain there permanently. A small tap on the exposed end is used to connect the dialysis fluid reservoir.

Two types of peritoneal dialysis are available: intermittent and continuous. Intermittent dialysis involves the use of a machine which pumps a large volume of fluid through the abdomen three or four times a week. The patient connects the catheter to the tubing of the machine, and dialysis lasts between ten and fourteen hours.

For continuous dialysis, fluid is run into the abdomen, left for several hours, removed, and replaced with fresh fluid. Usually the fluid is changed three or four times a day. Between fluid

Hemodialysis can be carried out successfully on all age groups. Those too young to dialyze themselves, or for whom home dialysis proves impractical, need to visit the hospital two or three times a week. The

alternative is a transplant operation. The baby (bottom) is being comforted by his parents after such an operation, while his grandfather looks on. The donor was the baby's mother.

Hospital meals are monitored to ensure that patients receive foods consistent with their treatment (right). Renal dietary requirements most often involve the regulation of protein and fluid intake.

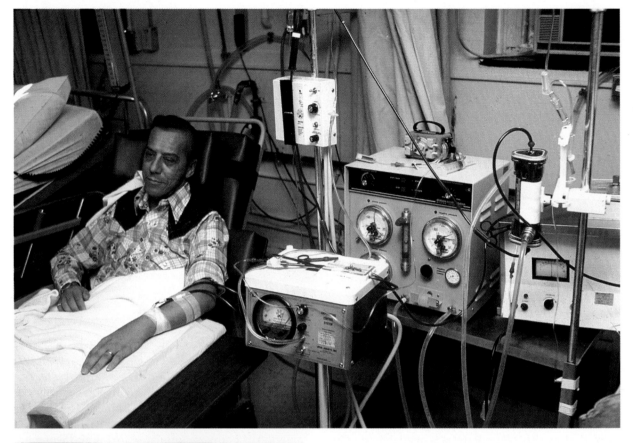

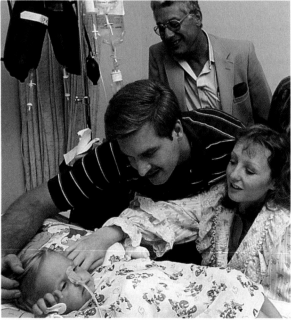

changes the patient is not connected to any machinery — although dialysis continues internally — and is therefore free to carry on with normal activities. For this reason the method is commonly known as continuous ambulatory peritoneal dialysis, or CAPD.

So what are the advantages and disadvantages of hemodialysis, and how does it compare with peritoneal dialysis? Hemodialysis is the more complicated technique and is limited by the number of sites available on the body to insert shunts or form fistulas. Some people find the machine formidable and cannot cope with their dependence on this "mechanical monster." Hemodialysis is still the most efficient way of removing wastes, but sometimes it can be too efficient and leave the patient feeling "washed out" for a day or so after treatment. If the dialysis removes too much water from the blood, blood pressure falls and the patient suffers from dizziness

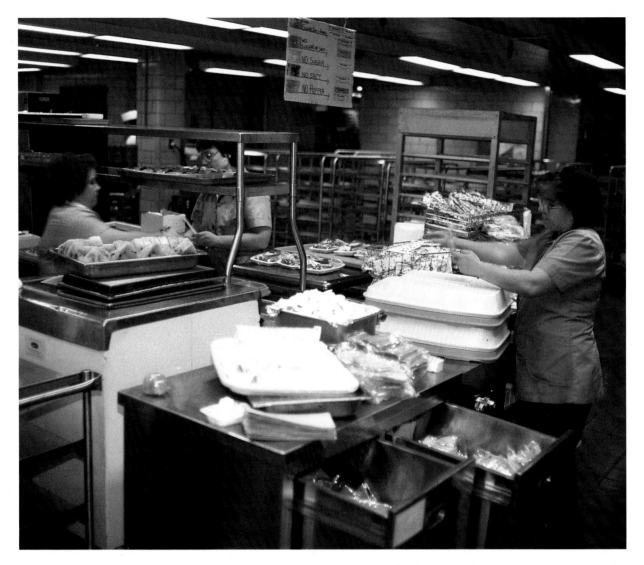

and fainting after being dialyzed. It is technically more complicated, and takes longer to learn, and the routine is not only hard to master but also requires at least one devoted helper.

Intermittent peritoneal dialysis overcomes a great many of these problems. It is simpler to learn and gentler in its waste removal. The fact that it is less efficient is a positive advantage, because a person does not run the risk of being "washed out." The entry to the patient's body is easier to make, too. Instead of the troublesome process of inserting a shunt or creating a fistula the patient can have the catheter inserted during a short overnight visit to a hospital or dialysis center.

IPD is not the ultimate answer for everyone, however. It is much slower than CAPD and a person must undergo thirty-six to forty-eight hours of dialysis a week. It still involves a machine, which can be just as restricting as the hemodialysis machine. It takes up about the same amount of space in the home and a person must go to the machine and stay there during dialysis. But IPD is valuable for patients who have problems with vascular access (especially those over sixty years old) and patients suffering from diabetes, because vascular disease is common with this disorder. Many people find the IPD apparatus far less threatening because there is no blood circulating through visible tubes, and they can make a better psychological adjustment to the trauma of being attached to a machine.

Continuous ambulatory peritoneal dialysis would seem the ideal solution. It involves gentle dialysis, simple equipment and lower costs. Patients on CAPD are allowed a more generous diet and need fewer or no drugs. In addition, many people on CAPD seem to have less trouble with anemia, a common symptom following kidney failure, and they describe themselves as suffering fewer symptoms in general. So why do some

Sir William Bowman

Revealing the Renal Function

In his lifetime, Sir William Bowman was probably better known as an ophthalmic surgeon of considerable ability than as a pioneer histologist (a specialist in the minute structure of tissues). Yet it is in the latter capacity that he is more famous today. Certainly, parts of the eye and tissues around the eye are known as Bowman's lamina and Bowman's muscle, but there is also Bowman's probe (for the examination of nasal ducts) and, above all, Bowman's capsule, part of the kidney.

Bowman was born in Nantwich, Cheshire, in England, in July 1816. After being apprenticed to a surgeon in the Midlands city of Birmingham, Bowman went south to London University and took up a minor post at King's College in 1837. Three years later he became assistant surgeon in the newly-established King's College Hospital (now one of London's most famous medical foundations). Although elected a Fellow of the Royal College of Surgeons in 1844, it was not until 1856 that his promotion to full surgeon at King's College Hospital was ratified, by which time he had become assistant surgeon (1846) and then full surgeon (1851) at the prestigious but more specialist Moorfields Ophthalmic

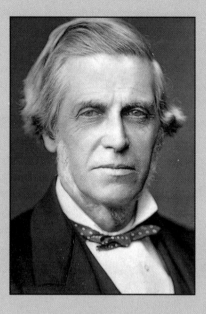

Hospital, also in London. He became a baronet in 1884.

Most of Bowman's discoveries about the functions of the kidneys were made in the early 1840s. Until that time it had not been established how urine formed and was passed out of the kidney through the ureter. Bowman was the first to grasp that the little vessel (capsule) enclosing each individual bunched group of blood capillaries (each glomerulus) in the nephrons was related to—and formed a terminus in—a single continuous tube (the renal duct), which eventually drains urine down into the bladder. The glomeruli were thus revealed to be part of a filtration system—a notion on which all succeeding views of kidney function are based. These findings were reported to the Royal Society in a paper entitled *On the Structure and Use of the Malpighian Bodies of the Kidney* in 1842.

A number of other discoveries of this kind were made public in a five-volume series of textbooks called *The Physiological Anatomy and Physiology of Man*, issued between 1845 and 1856 under his name and that of the contemporarily more eminent Professor at King's College, Robert Bentley Todd (1809–1860), Bowman's teacher and colleague.

Bowman finally became Professor of Physiology and General and Morbid Anatomy at King's College in 1848, by which time his fame as an ophthalmologist was nationwide. The first again to describe several optical functions and structures, he also introduced the clinical use of the ophthalmoscope (at which he was himself expert) and the surgical operation to remove the iris in the treatment of glaucoma.

A man of kindly reputation, a popular practitioner and an inspiring and innovative teacher, Sir William Bowman died in March 1892 in the town of Dorking, just south of London.

The disruptive routine of frequent hospital visits can be avoided by patients motivated to dialyze themselves at home, and who have a friend willing to learn and assist in the procedure. Self help often restores a sense of independence to patients who would otherwise feel overwhelmed by their condition and, because dialysis can be done during the night, their days can remain relatively undisturbed.

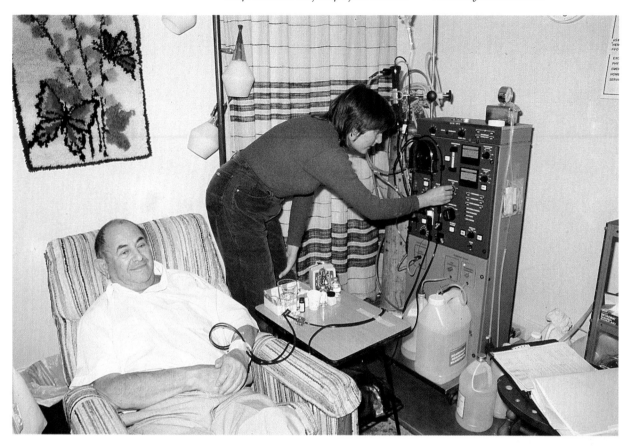

patients hemodialyze and others stay with IPD when CAPD seems to offer the perfect treatment?

The great drawback to CAPD is the risk of infection. Because the dialysis is continuous, the fluid must be changed three or four times a day. The technique involved is simpler than hemodialysis, but is still a boring routine that must be rigidly adhered to. The person must find a quiet corner, unfold a bag, attach a tube to the catheter and allow the fluid to run out of the abdomen. Then a new bag of fluid must be attached and fresh fluid run in. Rigid precautions are necessary to prevent bacteria, which will grow prolifically in dialysis fluid, from getting in with each manipulation. Again and again fluid is being poured into a part of the body that usually has no connection with the outside world and CAPD requires three or four hours each day of tedious and meticulous routine.

Despite all this care to attention and detail, most users have at least one episode of infection a year when the peritoneum becomes inflamed (peritonitis). Hospital admission and antibiotic treatment can overcome each episode, but in the long term multiple bouts of peritonitis scar the peritoneum and makes CAPD impossible. Despite these problems CAPD remains the most palatable form of dialysis for many people. The whole process, with its simple, portable equipment and ease of mastery, makes a person feel more "humanized." Improved methods may make bouts of peritonitis a thing of the past and push CAPD into the forefront of dialysis treatment in the future.

Questions of Life or Death

In 1960, when chronic dialysis became possible, a whole new series of difficult ethical questions also appeared. Machines and trained staff were in short supply and many young people needed urgent treatment. Who could make or should make the agonizing decisions as to who should get it?

The development of the miniature portable kidney has given renal patients the prospect of even greater independence. Vacations of two to three weeks become possible, with dialysis taking place on site.

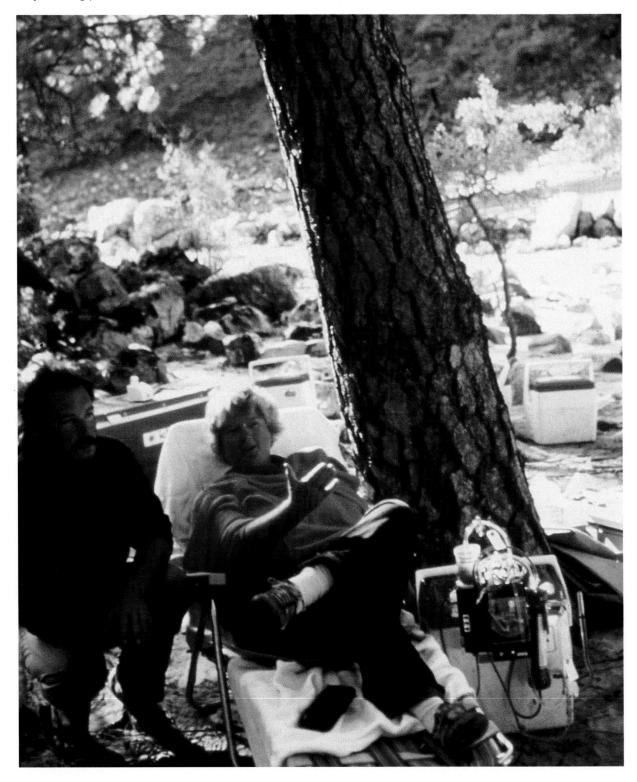

Within the few dialysis centers in existence, different methods of making the choice were decided upon. For example, some centers maintained a few highly trained renal physicians to make the decisions, whereas others adhered to a strict "first come, first served" rule. In Seattle, a unique panel of clergy, nonmedical and medical personnel were assembled to choose among the various candidates. An element of value to the community was made a criterion for life-saving treatment. But who really could decide between the relative merits of a young mother with children, and a single and talented scientist or musician?

Fortunately the number of hemodialysis centers increased rapidly and soon a rough balance between supply and demand developed. But this balance was still based on artificial factors. Only young people, usually those under the age of fifty, and people with relatively uncomplicated conditions were accepted. When it became clear that many patients, particularly diabetics, could benefit from dialysis, there was a great increase in demand for treatment and the inevitable question arose as to who should pay for this life-saving therapy. The more established a procedure dialysis became, the more stretched was the support from research funds. The cost of dialysis is about $25,000 per year for every person requiring it, and few people could afford this type of continuous outlay. Health insurance programs were reluctant to commit themselves to large sums which might continue for years, particularly because successful treatment resulted in long survival and an ever-increasing number of people needing treatment.

When Medicare and Medicard became national policy, an undesirable distinction occurred. People poor enough or old enough could have free dialysis, but everyone else was rationed. Congress had to step in and change the law to allow federal funding of all forms of treatment for everyone with end-stage renal disease. This major step toward federal involvement in health care may well be seen one day as the beginning of a National Health Service for the United States.

Kidney Transplants

Availability of efficient dialysis has been a major factor in the development of kidney transplanta-

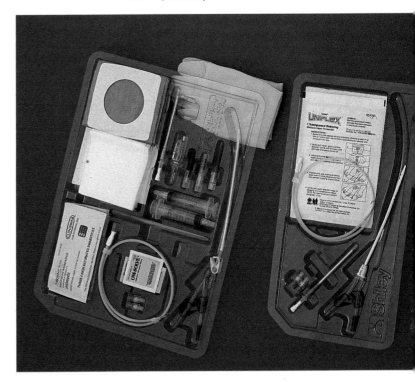

Once the basic technique of hemodialysis has been mastered, assembling the kits that accompany the portable kidney is quickly learned, using prepacked sterile needles (bottom).

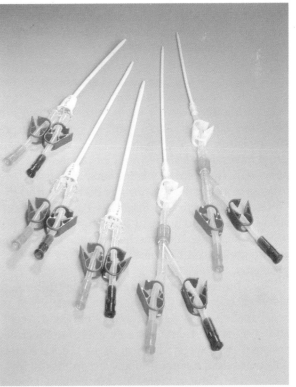

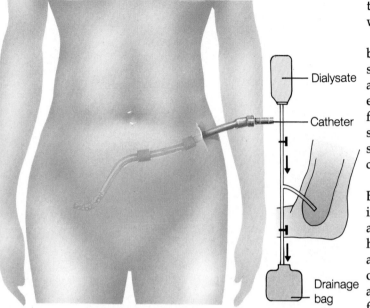

An alternative method of dialysis makes use of the body's own semipermeable membrane, the peritoneum. Dialysate is run into the abdominal cavity via a rubber catheter, which is left permanently inserted. Once toxins have been exchanged through the membrane, the fluid is drained away, the collecting bag emptied, and fresh dialysate is introduced into the patient's abdomen.

Dialysate

Catheter

Drainage bag

tion. If a person's kidneys fail, then he or she can be kept alive and well on dialysis while a suitable organ for transplantation is found. The importance of this is illustrated by the much slower development of the transplant programs for liver and cardiac replacement, caused in part by the inability to provide temporary mechanical replacement for these organs. Many potential recipients die before a suitable donor organ is found.

Unfortunately kidney transplantation does not hold the cure for every person suffering from kidney failure. If it did, then each person on dialysis could have a new kidney and their problems would be solved. The great barrier to transplantation is the process of rejection, in which the body destroys the "foreign" donor tissue. Rejection has been extensively studied and a few of the complexities of the process are now understood, enabling scientists and doctors to combat some, although not all, of the problems.

Each human body recognizes the difference between cells and tissues of itself and those of everyone else — the difference between "self" and "non-self." There is one exception to this rule, and that is between identical twins whose bodies see themselves as identical and accept tissue from each other. Indeed, some of the earliest kidney

transplants involved pairs of identical twins, one of whom had suffered from renal failure.

The basis for graft rejection is recognition by the body's immune system of complex proteins on the surface of normal cells, called histocompatibility antigens. These are inherited from parents and everyone therefore acquires one set of antigens from each parent. There is only a small chance that someone has the same antigens as a brother or sister, but there are at least some antigens in common with three out of four of siblings.

Early experiments by Sir Peter Medawar in Britain showed that transplant rejection was an immune response and involved both cells and antibodies of the immune system. Medawar and his colleagues Rupert Billingham and Leslie Brent also discovered that the immune system could occasionally be tricked into treating foreign tissue as "self." They showed that if mice are given a graft from a donor before birth they treat all other grafts from the same donor after birth as "self" and do not reject them.

This trick cannot be performed in humans because fetuses and newborn babies have more mature immune systems than mice. However, the idea that rejection could be prevented set off a great search for a clinically useful method to block the body's natural response.

Originally total body irradiation and large doses of steroid drugs were tried, but these were disappointingly ineffective. Clinical transplantation languished until 1960, when the drug azathroprine (Imuran) was introduced. After promising experiments in dogs by Professor R. Y. Calne (then at the Peter Bent Brigham Hospital in Boston and now at Cambridge, England), the drug was used in humans with hopeful results. Graft survival was prolonged from days and weeks to months in many cases. An explosion of interest and investigation followed. Could transplantation be made more successful and, if so, where would all the donor kidneys come from?

Transplants between identical twins were usually successful without much treatment, and so it seemed reasonable to use a close relative, usually a parent or sibling, as the donor. This is possible only because each of us has two kidneys and can get along perfectly well with only one of them. Also,

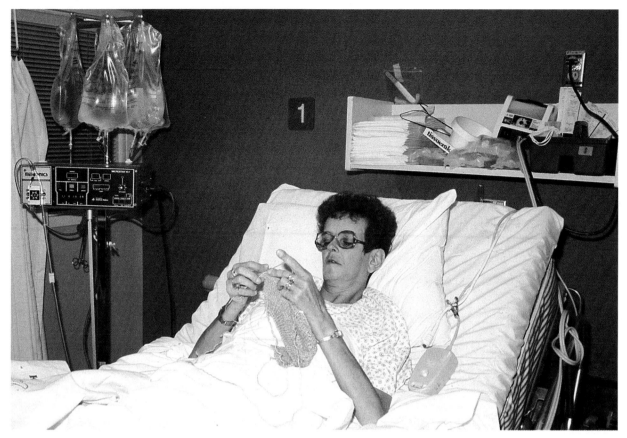

The efficiency with which hemodialysis removes wastes from the body can leave some people feeling "washed out," and is limited also by the number of sites available for introducing shunts or forming fistulas. Peritoneal dialysis (above) presents a more suitable alternative for patients with problems of vascular access and who need a gentler form of waste removal. Insertion of the catheter through the peritoneum, shown in section along the stomach wall (right), involves only an overnight stay in the hospital and does away with having to acquire the complex skill of "needling."

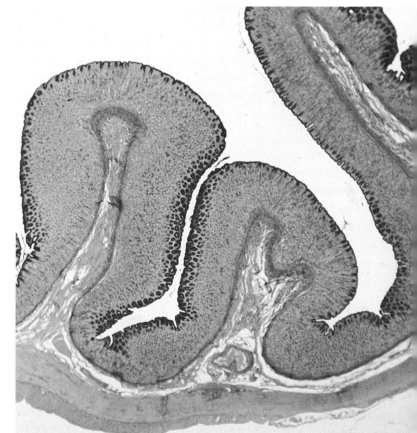

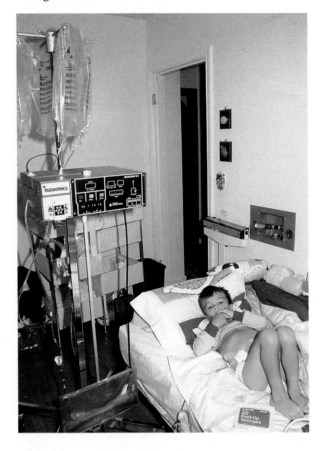

removing a kidney is a simple, safe operation so there is little risk to the donor. However, the important, and then unsolved, ethical issue was whether it was ever really justified to remove a healthy organ from someone when there was a chance that the transplant would fail.

One solution was to use kidneys from individuals who had recently died. Such "cadaver kidneys" could be successfully transplanted and function if removed within an hour or two of death. After this time, the organ is irreversibly damaged by the deterioration of the body. By itself the use of cadaver organs raised another group of ethical problems. Many potential donors were accident victims who had suffered severe brain damage and were being maintained on life-support machines. If medical opinion was that the victim was "brain dead" and had no chance of recovering consciousness or surviving off the respirator, was it permissible to switch off the machine? Who could make such decisions? And what was the definition of "brain death?"

The whole emotionally charged argument is made more spectacular by centers that had a "beating heart" cadaver program. All transplanted kidneys work better if the shortest time between death and reimplantation elapses, so after declaring a person "brain dead" the organs are removed before the life-support system is turned off. Indeed, this is now routine practice and it is the only way of obtaining heart or heart-lung grafts.

Obtaining consent to use organs is another difficult field of discussion. Which relatives have the right to make such a choice? If opinion is divided, how is the disagreement resolved? What, if any, rights does the intended donor have? It takes far too long to determine the contents of a will, which is therefore not the place to make final wishes about organ donation.

One solution is the donor card system. Anyone can carry a special card indicating that he or she would like to be an organ donor if possible. This does not completely eliminate the rights of the next of kin; but it does provide a strong indication of the potential donor's wishes.

But why do humans have to supply kidneys? Scientists use animal hormones to treat diabetes: why then do they not use monkey kidneys as an alternative source of transplantable organs? Unfortunately animal organs are rejected by the body by means of its powerful antibodies which rapidly destroy them by damaging the blood vessels. These antibodies are formed early in life — perhaps in response to bacterial infection — and there does not seem to be any way round this problem.

Antibodies and Antigens

Research has revealed that histocompatibility antigens are the target of rejection reactions in the body. The antigens were identified because some women formed antibodies to them when pregnant, and it was through the study of pregnant women that scientists found clues to the complicated process of rejection. After all, the fetus itself is made of tissue foreign to the body of the mother within which it is carried, so why is this "fetal graft" not rejected despite the presence in the mother's body of antibodies to the antigens of the fetus?

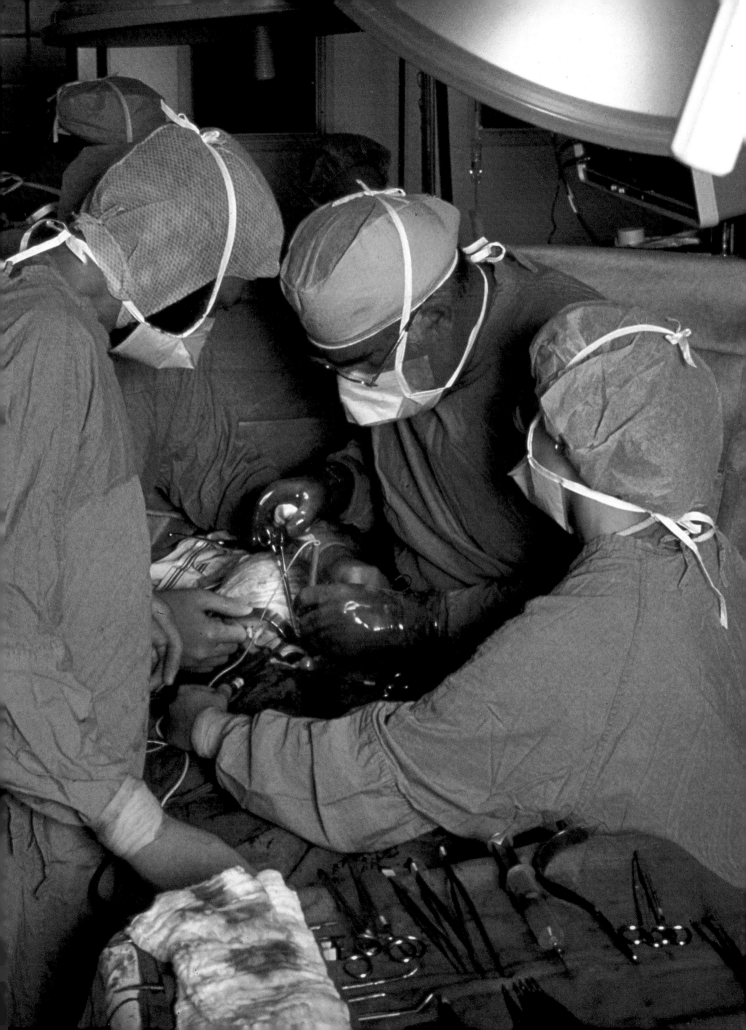

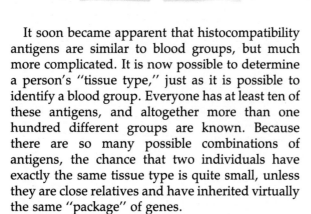

Nowadays it is not at all uncommon for a kidney to be transported hundreds of miles to be transplanted into a waiting recipient.

Reliable tissue typing has made it possible to set up a widespread transplant network, and this in turn has been greatly improved by a series of histocompatibility workshops held every three to four years. Initially, different laboratories used different antibodies, and there was no way to be sure how the results of two different places compared. A tissue type for a kidney obtained in one center might not mean the same thing as the tissue type of the potential recipient somewhere else. Techniques and antibodies have now been standardized so that any two laboratories register the same tissue type for the same single individual, and this uniform standard applies in most developed countries.

Widespread networks have also been made possible because kidneys can be stored for twenty-four hours or more, which enables them to be transported over longer distances. Once removed, the organ is filled with a chilled salt solution and packed in a sterile bag on ice. Even if it does not work perfectly the moment the transplant is complete, the recipient can be dialyzed for a few days while the transplanted kidney recovers full function. Often it is possible to tissue type a potential donor whose life is maintained on a respirator and search a computer file for the most compatible recipients, who are then notified to go to their nearest transplant hospital. When the donor dies, each kidney may be transported to a different destination.

Increasing Successes

The results of kidney transplantation improved steadily throughout the 1960s and 1970s. By the late 1970s the survival of all patients three years after receiving a kidney was about ninety per cent, and about half these people still had the same kidney. For those whose graft failed, further dialysis or a second, and sometimes even a third, transplant proved successful. Good results were partly because of better matching, but an unusual phenomenon also played an important part, which is now known as the "transfusion effect."

For a while during the early 1970s the success rate

It soon became apparent that histocompatibility antigens are similar to blood groups, but much more complicated. It is now possible to determine a person's "tissue type," just as it is possible to identify a blood group. Everyone has at least ten of these antigens, and altogether more than one hundred different groups are known. Because there are so many possible combinations of antigens, the chance that two individuals have exactly the same tissue type is quite small, unless they are close relatives and have inherited virtually the same "package" of genes.

Studies of many transplants showed that the more closely matched the tissue types of the donor and recipient, the longer the transplant survived. At first it seemed unlikely that a good "match" could occur unless close relatives were involved. Then eventually it was possible to collect enough information about a large number of people waiting for kidneys to enable the best match to be found for any particular donor kidney that became available.

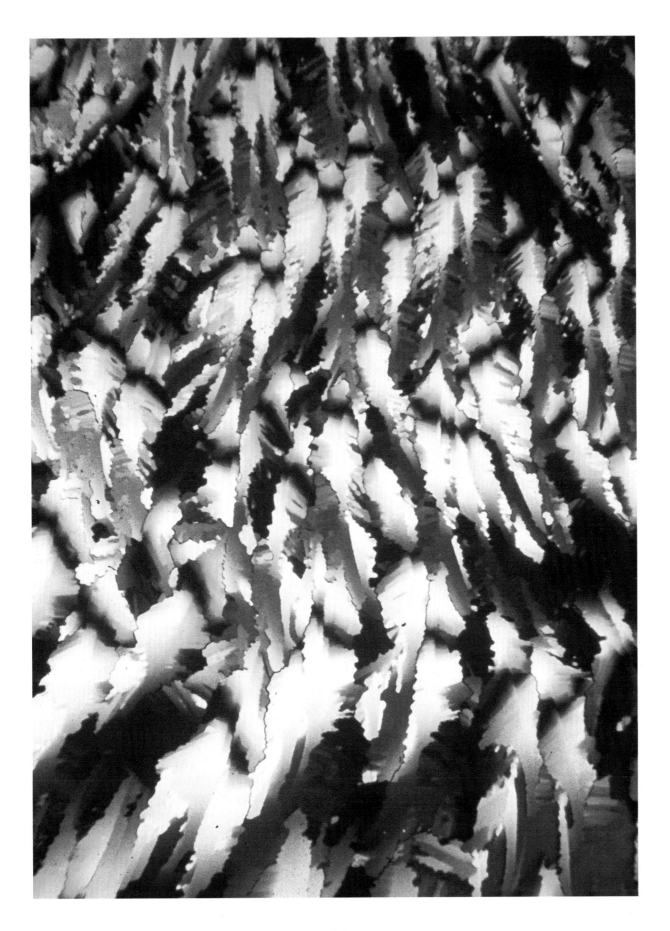

129

The immune system's recognition of complex proteins on the surface of cells, the histocompatibility antigens, is responsible for graft rejection. So far more than a hundred have been discovered, but because we inherit only eight from each parent, in two sets of four, there is a one in four chance that two siblings will share the same antigens and therefore easily accept transplant kidneys from each other.

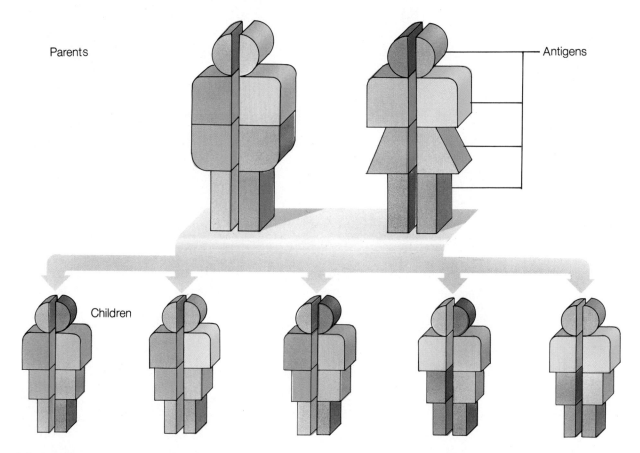

Parents

Antigens

Children

fell dramatically in many transplantation centers. After initial consternation and confusion, it was found that patients who had received blood transfusions before transplantation did very much better than people who had not received blood. This was noticed only because some dialysis patients had suffered from "hyperacute" rejection, having become sensitized by the numerous transfusions necessary to stabilize their condition.

Transfusions for dialysis patient are common for many reasons: anemia is a universal result of kidney failure; the artificial kidney machines in use in the 1960s required a "priming" volume of blood to start the pump working, and this was equivalent to a transfusion because the blood was from a blood donor rather than the patient. Some patients became sensitized and formed antibodies, which made their bodies reject any transplant very rapidly. To combat this an effort was made to eliminate all transfusions before transplantation.

Instead of an improvement in the success rate, the figures rapidly declined and scientists and doctors realized that in some mysterious way transfused blood inhibited the immune response against the transplant in the patients that did not suffer from hyperacute rejection. In complete contrast, many patients now awaiting grafts are deliberately transfused to produce this effect.

Until the late 1970s the drugs used to prevent graft rejection were usually Imuran and a type of steroid. Sophisticated ways of giving these agents were devised in an attempt to reduce their side effects. The chief culprit in the side-effect scenario was the steroid, which produced many life-threatening complications such as a risk of infections and perforated ulcers. Steroids can also produce death within the bone tissue itself, and many patients had to have artificial hip joints inserted to overcome the loss of bone. Steroids also inhibit growth, so that children who received a

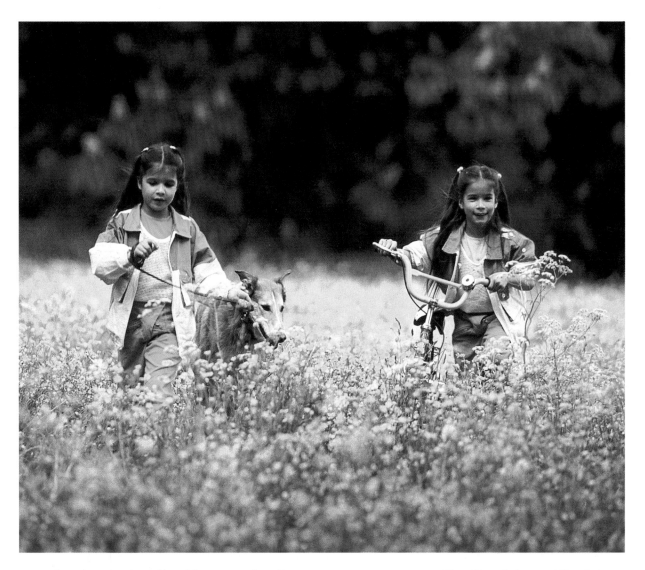

transplant frequently suffered from stunting. Every effort was made to keep the dose of steroids as low as possible, but occasional "rejection episodes" — sudden severe crises when the immune response to the graft became intense — called for high doses to combat the threat to the graft. These made the patient vulnerable to the side effects.

Then in the late 1970s a new agent, Cyclosporin A, revolutionized transplantation. Introduced by Professor R. Y. Calne of Cambridge and discovered by Dr Y. Borel of Sandoz Pharmaceuticals, this drug has dramatically altered the outcome of organ grafting. Cyclosporin A is an immunosuppressive agent, but its exact mode of action is still a mystery. It was discovered by chance and it seems remarkable that such a valuable agent should turn up so unexpectedly.

Cyclosporin has allowed physicians to prescribe steroids sparingly, or not at all in some cases. As a result, the complications they cause are greatly

The cells and tissues of identical twins are exactly matched so that, in comparing the two types, their immune systems do not differentiate between "self" and "non-self." For this reason, the earliest successful operations involved transplants using identical twins.

Donor kidneys can be preserved for twenty-four hours before they start to deteriorate. Filled with a special chilled salt solution, they are kept in sterile conditions prior to transplantation.

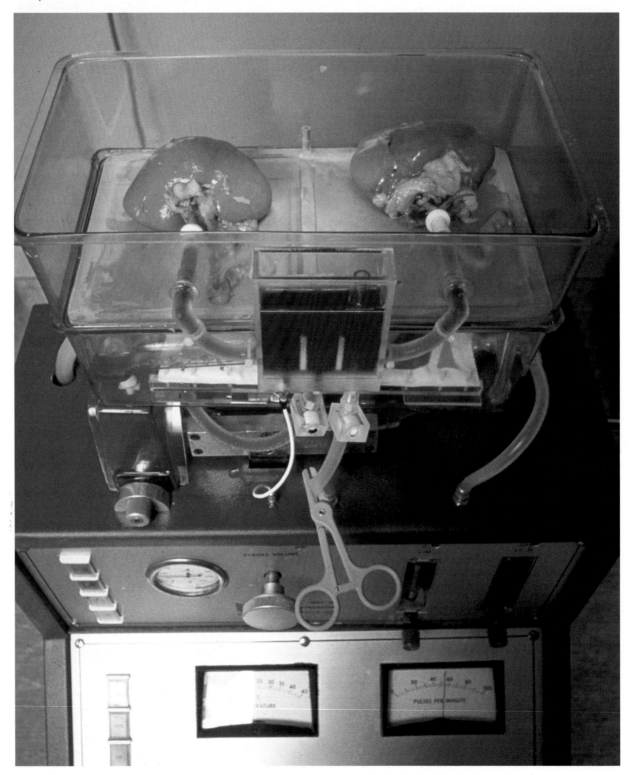

Reliable tissue typing has enabled a large transplant network to be set up between centers across the world. Computer technology (bottom) has made access to information about suitable donors more rapid still.

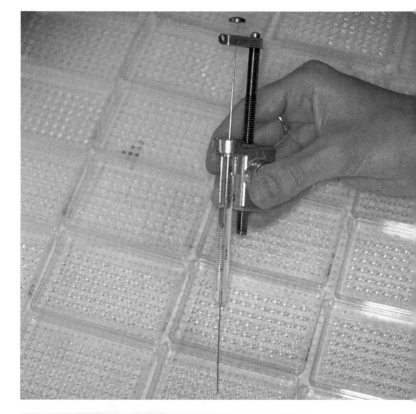

reduced. The side effects had often been so severe that steroid treatment had to be stopped and the graft was lost. So by decreasing the need for steroids not only was the treatment made more pleasant for the patient, it also greatly improved the numbers of successful transplants. Cyclosporin seems to shift the balance of the body's immune mechanism in the direction of treating the graft as "self." How this happens is an even bigger mystery, but it does mean that after several months some patients require only small doses of drugs to retain their graft. It is a deescalating — as opposed to an escalating — dosage drug.

Demand and Supply

Cyclosporin may also alter the whole strategy of kidney transplantation. Until recently there was a marked difference in the success of kidneys from live related donors and those taken from cadavers. About ninety per cent of well-matched live donor organs were still functioning three years after transplantation, but only forty to fifty per cent of cadaver grafts were still going. Recent figures indicate that, following the advent of Cyclosporin, the success rate for cadaver transplants has risen so that it is virtually the same as that for live donor organs. This alters the equation by which people and their doctors plan their therapy for renal failure. One of the leading transplant surgeons, Dr T. E. Starzl of Pittsburgh, has recently stated that the use of live donor kidneys is no longer justified because there is no advantage to the recipient and a slight risk to the donor.

The higher success rate of transplants of cadaver organs means that their use will become increasingly common, but unfortunately only about ten per cent of all suitable organs are made available for use and many thousands of useful kidneys are lost. Already people waiting for a graft may spend many months or years on dialysis before a suitable organ becomes available. For some, with very unusual tissue types, the wait for a good match may be too long. As demand increases the problem can only get worse. While much publicity has been aimed at persuading the public to be more prepared to donate a loved one's organs, little real progress has been made. One difficult problem is the reluctance of the physicians treating a potential donor to ask

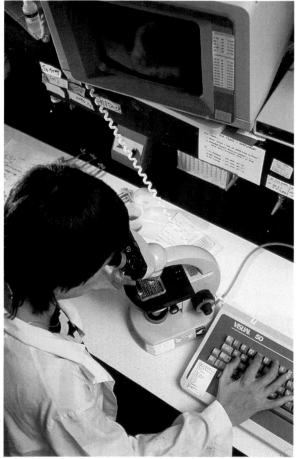

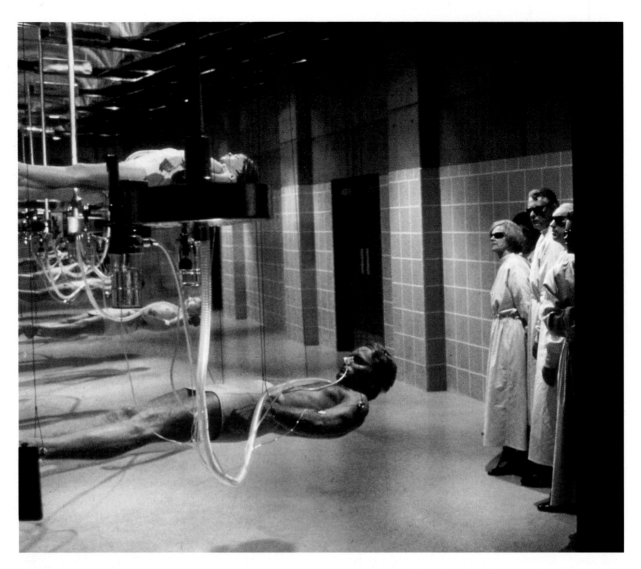

The use of cadaver kidneys has helped to alleviate the shortage of suitable organs for transplantation, but has also raised various ethical issues. Is it permissible, for instance, to turn off the life-support system of a potential donor who has no chance of regaining consciousness? Who should make that decision? The suspended, drugged, bodies in a scene from Coma (above) *play on the fear that healthy people might become unwitting donors in a ruthless method of "storing" transplant organs.*

permission of the already distressed relatives of a possibly tragic accident victim. Sometimes doctors are unaware of the great progress made in transplantation and feel that there is no point in obtaining organs. For the lay person it is often difficult to comprehend the difference between life and brain death.

The shortage of donor organs is so severe that many concerned individuals have begun to argue for a change in the law relating to organ procurement. Instead of an "opting in" system, which requires permission, an "opting out" system has been suggested. People would have to give written proof that they did not want their organs used after their death and, unless they did so, the law would presume that a person had no objection during life. Whether the public would accept such a change is questionable. Would there be a severe reaction to the image of bodysnatching? Perhaps relatives would sue, claiming that the deceased had

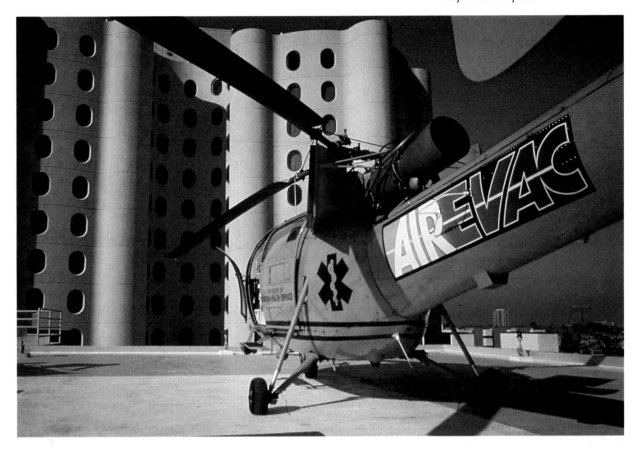

not been given optimum care because his organs were needed. Transplantation might even fall into disrepute. Understandably there is considerable reluctance to change laws if the end result could be detrimental to the very individuals the change should have benefited, and if the whole image of medicine as a caring patient-oriented profession might be jeopardized.

The Choices Now

Most people who develop chronic renal failure do so gradually over a period ranging from a few months to several years. This allows plenty of time for planning exactly which of the treatment options are most suitable, and a person has a chance to adjust to them.

Almost every renal failure patient starts on one form of dialysis or another. As we have seen, no form of treatment is clearly superior to all the others, and each person has unique requirements and resources which help to dictate his or her own choice. For example, although it is a relatively new method, CAPD seems very suitable for children because it allows greater freedom in the child's diet and in the amount of liquid consumed. Both of these are restricted on intermittent forms of dialysis. Furthermore, some of the side effects of renal failure, such as anemia, are less of a problem, and most children have parents who can help them with the daily dialysis routine.

For others there is the choice of either home or treatment-centered hemodialysis or intermittent peritoneal dialysis. Another factor that influences these decisions is the length of time for which dialysis is going to be necessary. If a histocompatible sibling is prepared to donate a kidney, then this attractive option means that dialysis is a temporary therapy. A patient without a suitable donor and an uncommon tissue type may be choosing a treatment he or she is to have possibly for life.

Before the development of the artificial kidney, some soldiers would be saved by a blood transfusion in the field, but die a few days later from acute renal failure caused by their initial loss of blood.

In the late 1970s the introduction of the immunosuppressive agent Cyclosporin, whose structure is shown (right), dramatically improved the success rate of cadaver kidney transplants.

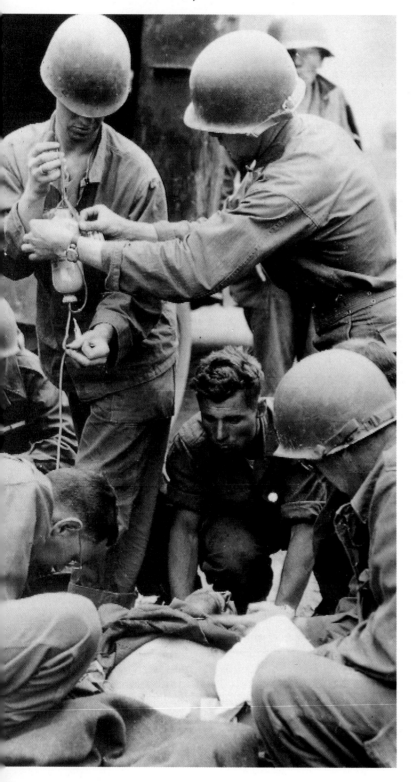

Unquestionably the best chance for rehabilitation of someone in renal failure is a successful transplant. After an initial period in the hospital for surgery and early immunosuppression, a person is discharged home and can shortly return to an essentially normal life. Indeed, the results of Cyclosporin treatment suggest that life will be very tolerable, with few long-term complications. Until recently, however, among cadaver transplants only about one recipient in three had an uncomplicated course with long-term graft function, and for many this was a disincentive to choosing the transplant option. Now that many centers are reporting that ninety per cent of their cadaver kidney recipients have functioning grafts two years after surgery, the balance is swinging in favor of transplantation. Furthermore, many people have had second and even third transplants successfully, so that the long-term prospect seems very promising. Even if a transplant fails after a few years, another graft extends a person's life — the clock is not irreversibly put back.

Overall, about half of all patients starting on dialysis will be alive three years later. About ninety per cent of related donor recipients and eighty per cent of unrelated donor recipients will survive this long too. There is, in addition, a continual year-by-year loss of people on dialysis as they move successfully onto transplantation, and for these people the major risk is over after the first few months — from then on survival is usually prolonged. This still leaves a gamble, a big risk leading to a better long-term outlook, but luckily this element of risk is being continually eroded by advances in the field of transplantation.

The Federal government applies a subtle financial pressure on the choice of treatment too, because it pays all costs for someone opting for home treatment or transplantation from the start, but pays for center-based treatment only after three months. Those three months can be expensive.

The Future

Nothing is ever so good that it cannot be better. Many strategies aimed at making transplantation foolproof are under investigation. Better tissue typing is being developed and several new antigens—which seem critical to graft rejection—

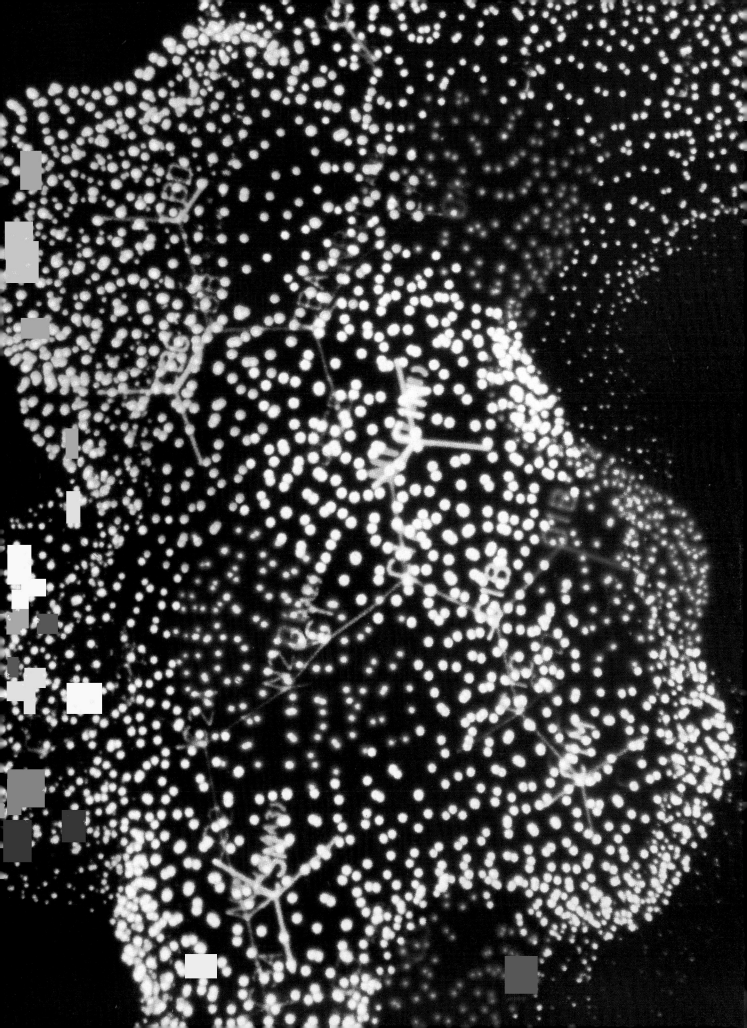

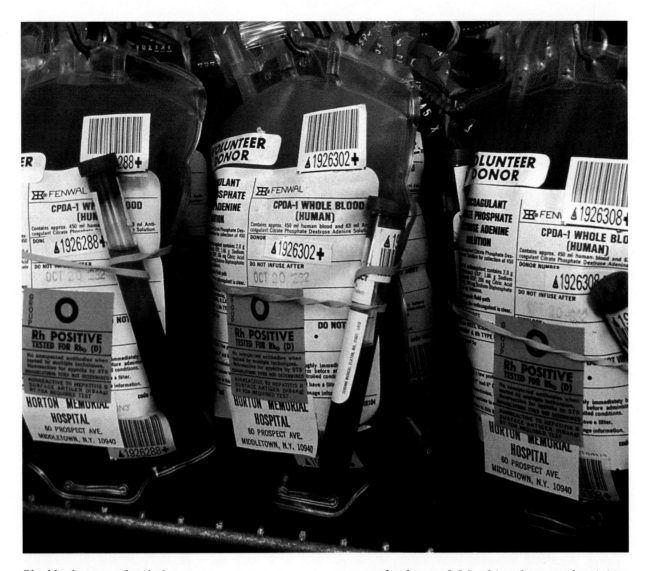

Blood banks ensure that the large amount of blood needed during many operations, including kidney transplantation, is readily available. A possible future step in renal research is the development of organ banks. Because at present donor kidneys can be stored for only twenty-four hours, a few are wasted and some go to moderately-matched recipients. Successful storage would enable a suitable kidney to be obtained and transplanted at exactly the right time.

can now be detected. Matching donor and recipient for these seems very promising. Several approaches to better immunosuppression are in the pipeline, and compounds similar to Cyclosporin A are being tested to see if they give even fewer side effects. Monoclonal antibodies have been developed which may selectively remove the white cells that cause rejection but leave untouched the body's defenses against infection. Exciting combinations of both drugs and antibodies seem possible, and perhaps one day it will be feasible to exploit the immunosuppressing effect of transfusions to pretreat people so that they are unlikely to reject grafts of certain tissue types. Such people would be immunologically engineered to treat particular foreign tissue as "self."

Ultimately, the increasing success of transplantation comes up against the barrier of organ supply. More efforts are being made to increase the number of kidneys available, and these must continue until enough potential donors exist to meet the foreseeable demand.

Another possibility for the future is the successful storage of kidneys. At present a few kidneys go to less well-matched recipients because they can be stored for only about twenty-four hours. If organ banks became feasible, they could become like blood transfusion banks and a suitably matched kidney could be stored for years if necessary and then retrieved from storage and transplanted at just the correct moment.

In the future, a major shortage of organs for transplantation may necessitate a review of the use of animal organs. At present such transplantations are not possible because of rejection problems. Perhaps a way could be found to surmount the species barrier and remove the cells of the recipient's antibodies that would destroy the graft. Alternatively, antibody production could be shut off long enough to let the transplant "take."

Preventing Kidney Failure

A major exciting prospect is the possibility that chronic renal failure may actually be preventable. In some people progress to renal failure is a slow, but certain, event. Recently it has become known that a failing kidney is further damaged by doing its normal filtering of waste and protein. Rather like the filter in a coffeepot, it becomes blocked up when used too often and, as the size of the available filter becomes smaller, the chances of the filter becoming blocked increases. It is the same with the kidney: the smaller the available area for filtration becomes, the more susceptible is the kidney to further deterioration because of blockage by the material it is filtering.

People in the early stages of renal deterioration may have the rate of their kidney damage slowed by important changes in their diet. At present the totally protein-free diet being tested is extremely unpalatable, but in time further research may develop an acceptable diet that has the same effect of reducing the load on the kidneys. Some patients may avoid the need for renal replacement altogether, although whether major dietary changes could become more acceptable than an improved prospect for successful transplantation is obviously still open to speculation.

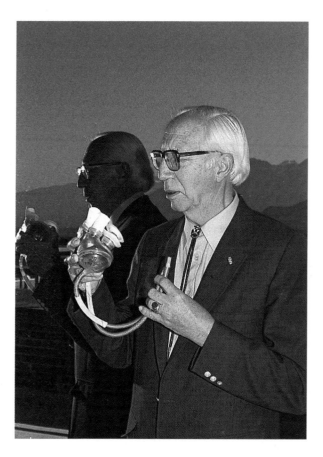

The kidney was the first organ in the body to have its chief function taken over by a machine. The machine's inventor, Willem Kolff, went on to use the experience he gained during its development to produce an artificial heart, which he is here seen holding.

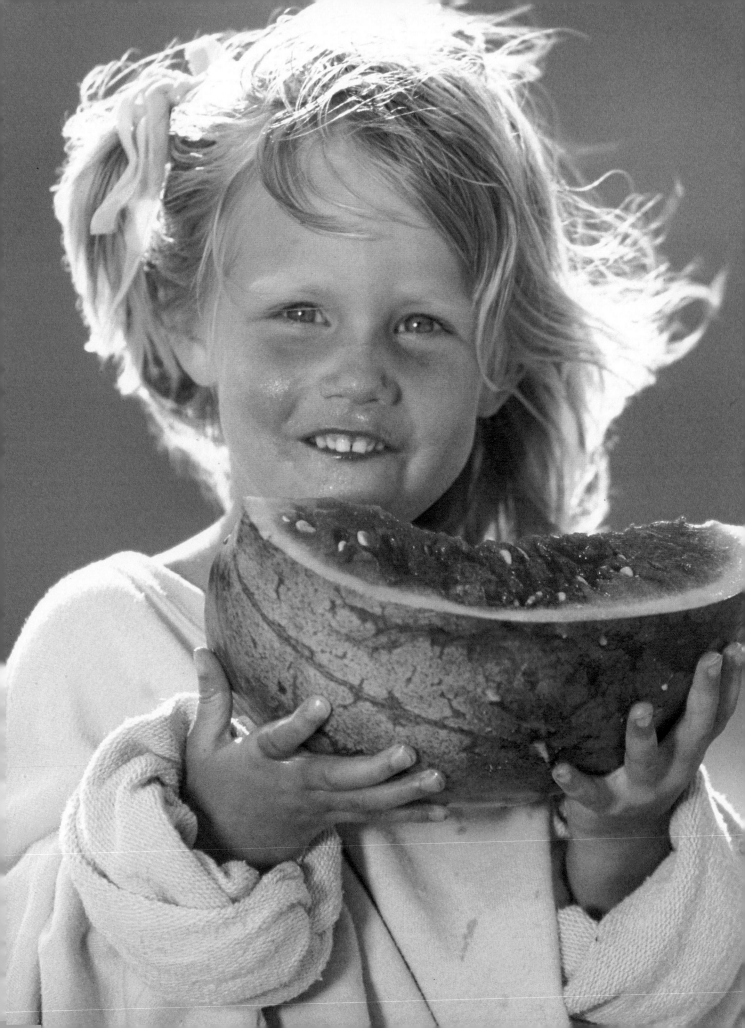

Chapter 6

Environmental Influences

The kidneys are paired organs in which no fewer than a million tiny tubules (nephrons) twist, bend, dip, ascend and finally drain down into the ureters. Through the tiny networks of glomeruli capillaries encircled by a Bowman's capsule at the head of each nephron, nearly forty-eight gallons of fluid are filtered each day, and yet only about half a gallon reaches the bladder through the ureters. Millions of years of evolution have gradually altered and molded the structure and functions of the mammalian kidney in order that it should meet the challenging demands of living on land.

When creatures first wriggled out of water onto land, a major problem they had to face was that of water conservation and of maintaining the right concentration (osmolality) of salts and other solutes in their body fluids. Before this they had been surrounded by an infinite volume of water which they "breathed," so their kidneys were primarily, if not solely, concerned with salt conservation. Living on land thus presented a new challenge—maintaining the overall fluid balance—and so the function, and thus structure, of the kidney had to evolve further if they were to survive and go on to reproduce their kind.

Evolution and Kidney Function

The first land creatures were amphibians which breathed through lungs yet used their skins as a source of water. Obliged to remain near ponds and lakes, their excursions on land were necessarily limited, for if water could be intaken through the skin it could also be lost through the skin. And they had no mechanism that told them when they were thirsty. But they did develop the ability to reabsorb much of the water content of the kidneys' output when they ventured farther afield. To accommodate this process the antidiuretic hormone probably evolved—a method of water conservation. From then on, as the vertebrates progressed through further evolutionary stages, water con-

Water constitutes a major part of our daily diet. It is consumed as fluid and in high-water-content foods such as fruit, often in greater quantities than the body requires. The kidney, however, is designed to permit this freedom of excess, allowing the human "machine" to take in more than it needs of many necessities—such as water and salt—and excreting what is not required.

141

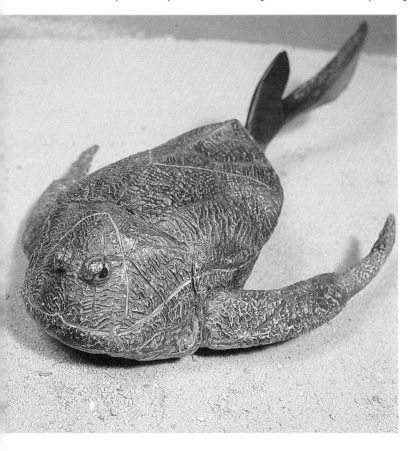

did — it was necessary for them to develop an excretory system from which the least possible amount of sodium and water were lost. Unlike mammals, which excrete their nitrogenous waste products in the form of urea in urine, reptiles and birds excrete uric acid. This molecule carries twice as much nitrogen as urea, and less water is required for its excretion. Furthermore, even in the cloaca — the final part of the alimentary canal — of birds and reptiles, water is absorbed and the uric acid precipitates out of solution; only a whitish sludge is actually excreted. The excretion of uric acid thus represents a water-conserving device of great efficiency, and because only a small amount of concentrated urine is produced, the networks of glomeruli in the kidneys of reptiles and birds are small and the filtration rate is slow.

Mammals also need to conserve water, and they therefore excrete urine which is more concentrated than their body fluids. However, mammals (and birds) have an internal "thermostat" which enables them to regulate their own body temperature irrespective of the external environment — they are homeotherms — and as a consequence the rate at which food substances are metabolized has to be relatively high to generate the necessary heat. To sustain such a metabolic rate a high rate of blood flow, and a correspondingly high blood pressure, is required. This high pressure means that large quantities of fluid are forced through the glomerular filters into the nephrons. Nearly all of this fluid — as much as ninety-nine per cent — is reabsorbed later.

The device for the concentration of waste material as evolved in mammals does not involve the excretion of uric acid — in fact mammals excrete urea like their aquatic and amphibian ancestors. What mammals developed were very long nephrons encompassing a long loop, the loop of Henle. This provides a counter-current system which, as explained elsewhere, creates an osmotic gradient from the cortex to the medulla of the kidney. Water can be reabsorbed, and concentrated urine produced. In fact the length of the U-shaped loop of Henle directly relates to the need for water conservation in each specific mammal. Desert animals, for example, thus have relatively long loops of Henle and can therefore produce very

servation remained of primary importance; there was never any need for a diuretic hormone that would promote water loss.

The kidneys of amphibians are very similar to those of their ancestors the freshwater fish, but by the additional monitoring of the osmolality and sodium content of the body and the appropriate regulation of these with antidiuretic hormone and aldosterone, the kidneys in their new form were able to combat the problems of maintaining a stable internal environment away from an aqueous external environment.

Reptiles and birds represent the final escape from a watery habitat. In reptiles the permeable skin of the amphibian is replaced by impermeable scales; birds too may be regarded as basically no more than feathered reptiles. The only way for these two great classes of animals to obtain salt and water is to eat and drink. Accordingly, for them to invade relatively dry habitats — as indeed the dinosaurs

In command of both excretion and osmoregulation, the nephron can be regarded as the functional unit of the kidney. Blood flowing through the kidney is first conveyed to the nephron's glomerulus, where blood *containing salts, urea and water filters into the hollow Bowman's capsule. This passes into the proximal convoluted tubule, where salts, glucose and water are reabsorbed into the blood. Urine is* *concentrated when it reaches the loop of Henle by the absorbtion of more water into the blood against an osmotic gradient. This osmotic pressure keeps urine at about the same concentration as blood.*

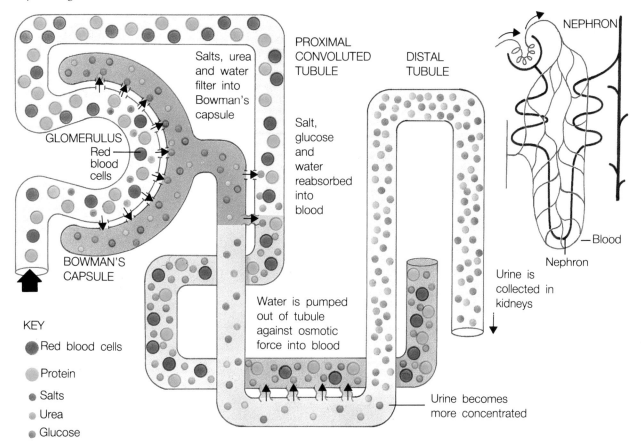

concentrated urine, and as a consequence they suffer only a minimal water loss.

Special Requirements of Humans

Humans are less tolerant of water shortage than most land creatures. The maximum weight loss due to desiccation that a person can survive is about twenty per cent of normal body weight. On the other hand, rodents such as rats and mice can withstand up to thirty per cent body weight loss, and cats can lose up to forty per cent of their body weight of water. The earthworm is even more remarkable; as it wriggles through the soil it is able to tolerate a loss of well over half of its body weight — up to sixty per cent in fact — through desiccation. Birds and reptiles can lose up to fifty per cent. In fact, the rate at which an animal becomes dehydrated is just as important as the degree of dehydration. For example, if a frog becomes dehydrated slowly it can survive a forty per cent reduction in body weight; but if the dehydration occurs rapidly, only a twelve per cent loss in body weight is tolerated before the dehydration becomes lethal.

For humans, the maximum survival time without water is between eleven and twenty days, provided that favorable conditions (including shade and a moderate environmental temperature) are available. A person stranded in the desert under direct sunlight can survive for only a matter of hours. Under such conditions more than two pints of water may be lost as sweat each hour, representing no less than about one-twelfth of the total extracellular water normally contained within the human body.

At a water deficit of about three per cent body weight, salivary secretions and urine volume diminish. Even if that deficit rises to five per cent, no serious disturbances occur, although the heart rate and body temperature may increase and a

The patches of familiar white guano that embellish the rocks of cliff-tops are a certain indicator that large numbers of birds are nesting nearby. This nitrogenous waste product, containing uric acid, results from the breakdown of protein during digestion. Requiring less water than urea does for its excretion, uric acid is also excreted by reptiles and, through a quirk of breeding, by Dalmatian dogs.

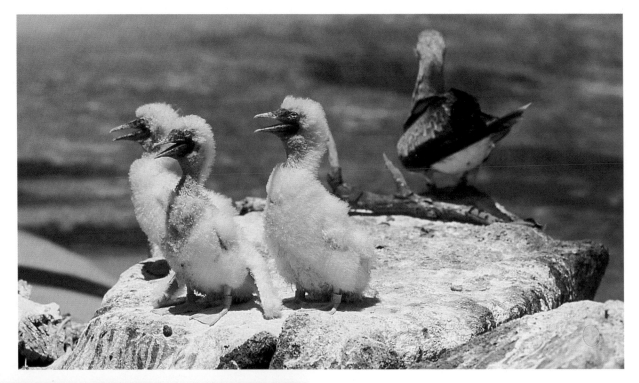

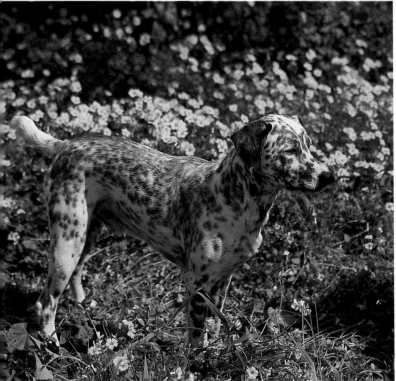

certain degree of lassitude may be felt (this can happen in a hot climate without dehydration). When the loss of body weight exceeds ten per cent, however, there is a dramatic weakness, a reduction in physical strength and a failure of some mental powers. By the time a twelve per cent loss is reached, swallowing becomes impossible. Depending on the rapidity of dehydration and climatic conditions, death occurs when the human body has lost between fifteen and twenty per cent of its weight in water. No one really knows the actual final cause of a death due to desiccation although, clearly, there is failure of the blood circulation because of loss of plasma volume and increase in the blood viscosity. Another possible factor is cellular death, caused by the high concentration of salt in the water-depleted body fluids.

Infants are even more susceptible to dehydration. A child weighing eleven pounds contains almost one gallon of body water, and a normal daily fluid intake of about one and a half pints thus corresponds to about one-quarter of total body water — and one-half of extracellular fluid. In contrast, the average adult intake is about four

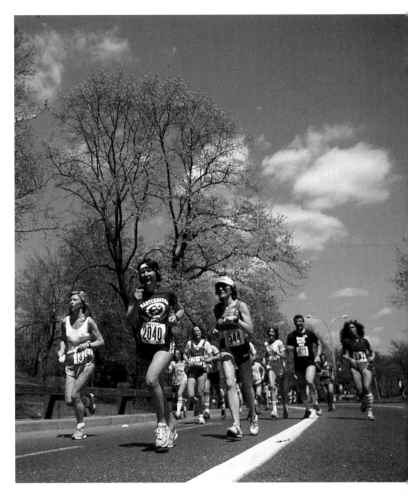

pints a day, a quantity of fluid that corresponds to only about five per cent of total body water or fifteen per cent of extracellular fluid. Excessive water loss in a child, therefore — whether due to vomiting, diarrhea or sweating — leads to a serious degree of dehydration about five times more quickly than in an adult.

The Thirsty Castaway

A person on a raft at sea, or stranded on an island without fresh water, is in as difficult a situation as the unfortunate individual stranded in the desert. The salt content of the large oceans may be as high as three and a half per cent but the human kidney cannot excrete urine with a salt content greater than two per cent. So for every cupful of seawater that the shipwrecked sailor drinks, one and three-quarter cupfuls of urine must later be passed in order to get rid of the excess salt consumed. And passing that quantity of urine merely worsens the problem of dehydration and induces an even greater thirst. (Everyone knows that it only takes eating a few ''salty'' snacks to bring on quite a thirst.) Furthermore, the magnesium content of the sea promotes diarrhea, which in turn leads to further water loss. In fact, the only benefit a castaway can derive from the sea is by wetting the skin or clothes with water for coolness. In this way the need for profuse sweating is limited.

Experience has shown that an ignorant castaway who drinks seawater dies more quickly than the more informed shipwrecked sailor who resists the temptation. Nevertheless, there are reports — and, indeed evidence — that drinking seawater can have life-saving value. First, certain seas such as the Black Sea and the Caspian Sea have only half the salinity of the Atlantic Ocean; some parts of the Baltic Sea have almost the same salinity as the body fluids. Although concentrated, some water could be extracted and absorbed from urine deriving from these sources. Second, in hot climatic conditions salt losses from the body resulting from sweating are so acute that drinking small amounts of seawater to replace the lost salt are actually beneficial. (This is the case only when normal rations of fresh drinking water are simultaneously available.)

So, unless you are shipwrecked in a sea containing a low proportion of salt, do not drink the seawater. But can you eat the fish that have jumped onto the raft or been caught in a makeshift net? The answer is again that you should not. Once more, you would need to pass as urine all the water content of the fish in order to excrete the salt and protein contained in it. The problem of dehydration is not solved — pray for rescue instead.

Water Balance

Being castaway on a raft or sitting on a desert island in company with a solitary palm tree is not a common occurrence, although the scenario has been widely used as an ideal situation to illustrate the problems of water balance. A more realistic situation is presented by modern equipment provided for occupants of lifeboats and life-rafts where the availability of fresh water may become a life-saving necessity. Several methods of extracting fresh water from seawater have been developed. Some rely on distillation, using the heat of the sun, but distilling apparatus is complex and bulky, and hardly suitable for incorporating into the life-saving packs of lifeboats. In preference, chemical methods

Like rows of miniature icebergs, salt deposits form from evaporating of brine. Forty million tons of salt are produced in the United States every year; this chemical in the diet is essential for health.

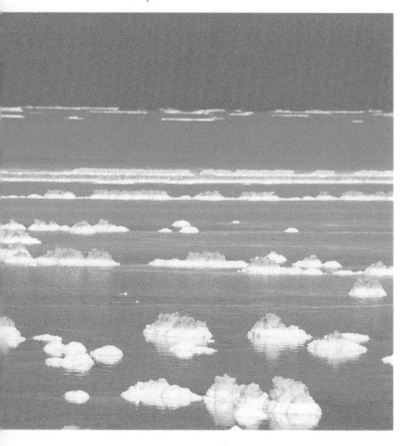

of purification are now widely used, based on the principle of chemically precipitating most of the salt out of the seawater.

The development of chemical procedures has been greatly simplified by two facts. First, water containing about 0.3 to 0.4 per cent of salt actually tastes much better than pure distilled water containing no salt. It is also better suited to the body's needs and results in greater water conservation because the reabsorbtion of salts leads to the reabsorbtion of proportionately more water. Second, the sulfate contained in seawater is harmless to humans.

An adequate supply of water is thus essential for survival — and although salt is necessary to maintain the correct distribution and volume of body fluids, the body is able to stay in "sodium balance" on a diet virtually free of salt. If salt is restricted the body fluid may initially shrink by a considerable amount, but afterward a new steady state of the extracellular fluid is reached and virtually no salt is excreted. No steady state is reached when water supplies are severely restricted or entirely absent.

Some animals have adapted to the most adverse of external environments, such as the deserts and marine environments, both of which are hostile to human survival. How do they manage to regulate their internal environment, to obtain sufficient salts and water, and to excrete the waste products of their metabolism?

The internal regulation of body fluids in desert animals is dominated by the most urgent need to conserve water. All mammals gain water by eating and drinking; some desert animals — such as the kangaroo rat (*Dipodomys* spp) — are entirely dependent on their food for their water supplies. Even apparently dry food such as grain may contain between twenty and thirty per cent water, and when the food substances are broken down, or oxidized, even more water and carbon dioxide are produced. The oxidation of fats and carbohydrates is useful in this respect, but the oxidation of protein produces not only water but also ammonia, urea or uric acid. These nitrogen-containing waste products must be excreted — and this by itself requires a loss of water which may be greater than the amount of water the protein has produced in the first place.

Water is lost mainly in urine, through respiration and by evaporation from the skin, and death by desiccation is prevented in desert animals by special adaptations to restrict these methods of water loss. For one thing, the kidneys of desert mammals have relatively long loops of Henle and so can produce urine that is highly concentrated — much more highly than any human's, for example. This means that less water is excreted by the kidneys.

Many animals also remain in microclimates in which the temperature is lower and the humidity higher than the surrounding air. Any crack or crevice, such as the space under a fallen leaf, is cooler and retains a higher humidity than the environment, and even the air in the interstices of apparently dry soil is usually saturated with water. Such a relatively cool microclimate reduces the need for heat loss and hence water evaporation

This unusual painting entitled **Water** by Giuseppe Arcimboldo, depicts a head created entirely from seafood. Eating food with such a high salt content produces an above average level of dissolved substances in the blood. The high blood concentration activates the secretion of antidiuretic hormone (ADH), which causes the reabsorbtion of water in the kidney tubules so that less urine is passed.

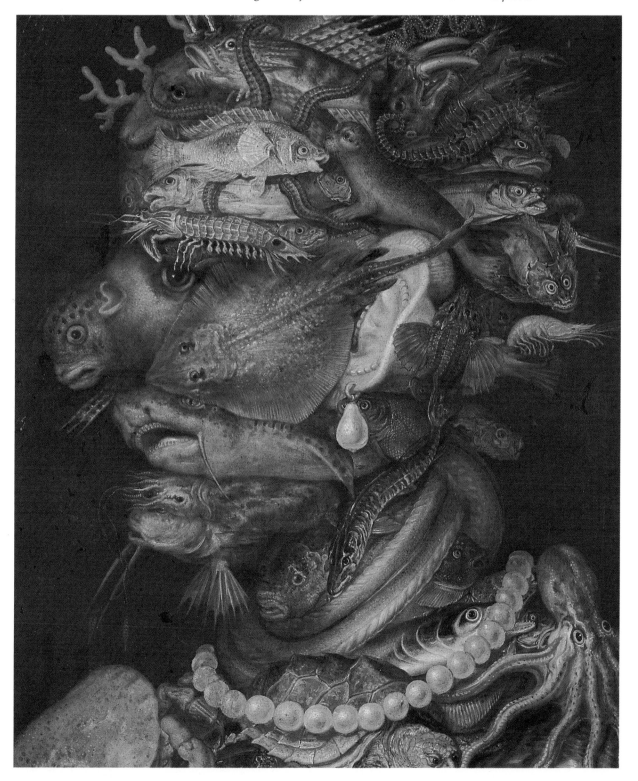

KIDNEY TUBULES IN VERTEBRATES

| Glomerulus

| Proximal tubule

| Distal tubule

| Loop of Henle

| Collecting duct

The length and complexity of vertebrate kidney tubules (below and bottom) is determined by the severity of the problems involved in controlling the amount of water and salt that enters and leaves the cells

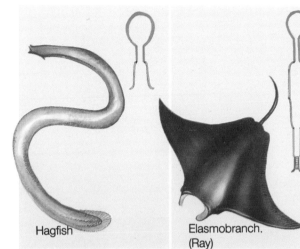
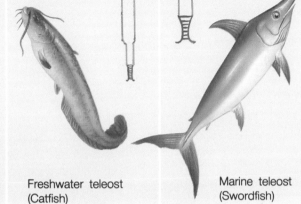

Hagfish

Elasmobranch. (Ray)

Freshwater teleost (Catfish)

Marine teleost (Swordfish)

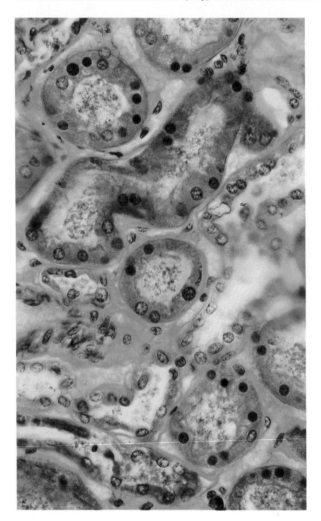

from the skin (thermoregulation). Higher humidity additionally serves to lower the loss by evaporation from both the skin and lungs. The North American kangaroo rat, for example, lives in burrows during the day where the humidity is high and the temperature is low. Provided that the humidity does not fall below twenty per cent, this animal can survive on a dry vegetable diet without actually drinking any water at all.

Another adaptation to the desert seen in the kangaroo rat is its ability to maintain a lower temperature in the skin lining its nasal passages than in its overall body temperature. Water in the warm, saturated air passing out of the lungs may thus condense on the relatively cool lining of the nasal passages, and in this way some of the water vapor lost from the lungs may be recovered. Quite how this animal cools the lining of its nasal passages is not known, but there must be some intricate yet extremely efficient heat-exchange mechanism.

The camel presents a somewhat different evolutionary answer. It cannot creep into a burrow nor hide under a fallen leaf in the heat of the midday sun. However, in times of water shortage it has several ways of reducing the amount of water lost through sweating. First, it simply allows its body temperature to rise so that sweating is not needed to keep the body temperature down. Second, the thick hair on the back reduces the effect of solar heat on the animal, while the thin hair

and body fluids. The composition of urine tends to mirror the water needs of the organism. The hagfish has blood as concentrated as seawater, and therefore little need for water regulation, so the nephrons are

short. Freshwater fishes usually excrete very dilute urine, an activity made possible by their large glomeruli. Marine bony fishes have small glomeruli which allow them to combat water loss in their salty

environments by excreting concentrated urine. In amphibians, reptiles, birds and mammals, an additional region appears in the kidney tubules — the loop of Henle — which operates to remove water.

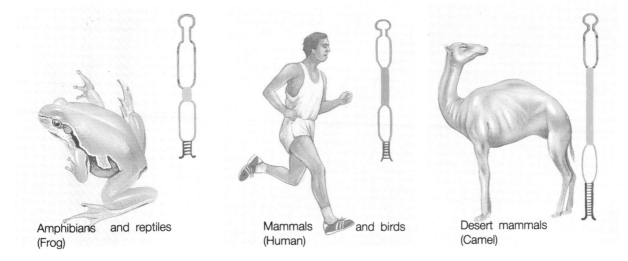

Amphibians and reptiles (Frog)

Mammals and birds (Human)

Desert mammals (Camel)

underneath helps heat loss. Third, much of the fat beneath the camel's skin is concentrated in its hump (which is not filled with water, despite the stories). Fat is a good insulator, and so if it is concentrated in one (or two) areas of the body rather than being evenly distributed over the entire body, a greater amount of heat can be more readily lost from those areas of the body that are not covered by it. This reduces the need to actively sweat in order to lose heat.

Finally, the camel has a very high tolerance to dehydration. It can lose more than thirteen gallons of water and yet its plasma volume is reduced by less than half a gallon. It has some mechanism by which blood volume is maintained despite a severe loss in the proportion of total body water. This adaptation circumvents, to some extent, the circulatory problems that would otherwise result from desiccation, and enables the camel to survive for at least seventeen days in tropical high summer without drinking; in winter it can go without water indefinitely.

Marine mammals, such as seals and whales, in some ways have a problem similar to that of the desert animals and of the shipwrecked sailor. It is likely that marine mammals do not drink any significant amount of seawater and that, similar to many desert animals, they rely wholly on their food as the source of water and salts. They do have an advantage, however, over their terrestrial relatives in that they do not have the same problems of

thermoregulation and loss of water by sweating. They also have an ability to extract a much greater proportion of oxygen from any specific quantity of air (which is why they can dive for long periods); less air is thus required to pass in and out of the lungs, and as a result less water is lost through respiration.

On the other hand, marine birds and reptiles do actually drink seawater. Many have evolved special nasal glands to secrete the excess salt ingested with the water. Some reptiles alternatively shed salty tears. (So "crocodile tears", in the biological sense, are merely an outward sign of internal salt and water regulation in these animals.)

The Challenge of Outer Space

The ultimate adaptation of animals, including humans, that might be envisaged for the future is one to the conditions of outer space. But manned flight to the moon, and possibly to planets such as Mars, poses a completely different situation in that in these environments there is simply neither water nor gravity.

The transport of large quantities of water to outer space is, contemporarily at least, out of the question. The only apparently practicable way out of this dilemma is thus to recover and recycle the water lost to each individual through the lungs, skin and kidneys. Among the most promising methods of reclaiming urinary water involves freeze-drying of urine, followed by its filtration

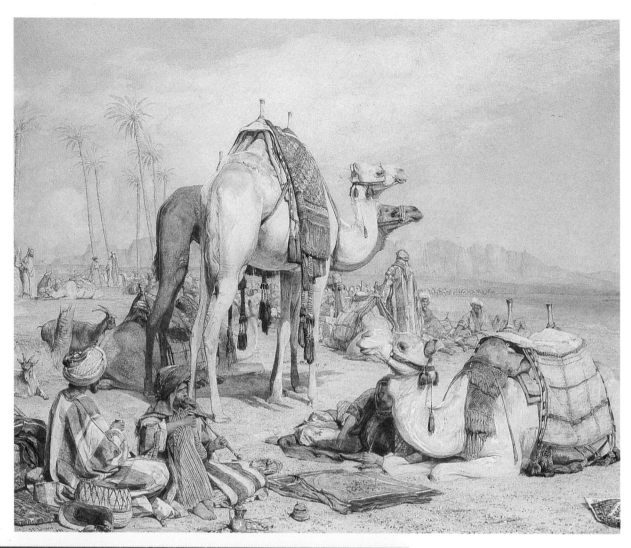

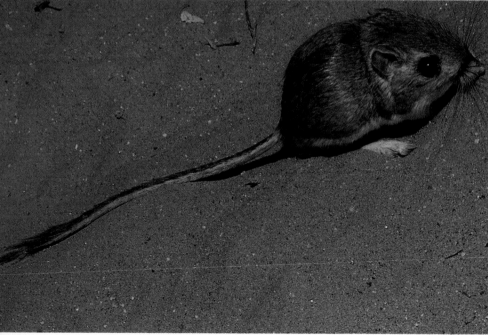

The camel and the kangaroo rat each has its own unique way of conserving water. Camels can go without drinking for many days, because they lose their body fluid very slowly, helped by the methods they employ to reduce the need to sweat. Camels can, however, regain lost fluid in as little as ten minutes by drinking up to 25 gallons of water. In contrast, the kangaroo rat rarely ever needs to drink water because it obtains most of the moisture it requires from its food. Because this animal lives in burrows where the humidity is high and the temperature low, it loses little moisture from the skin and lungs.

Early nursing staff were quick to recognize the importance of an adequate supply of drinking water in order to prevent dehydration. The most common cause of dehydration is failure to drink, which is potentially serious because humans lose about 2.5 per cent of their body fluids daily. Patients suffering from vomiting or diarrhea may need an extra pint or more of fluids a day to replace those lost.

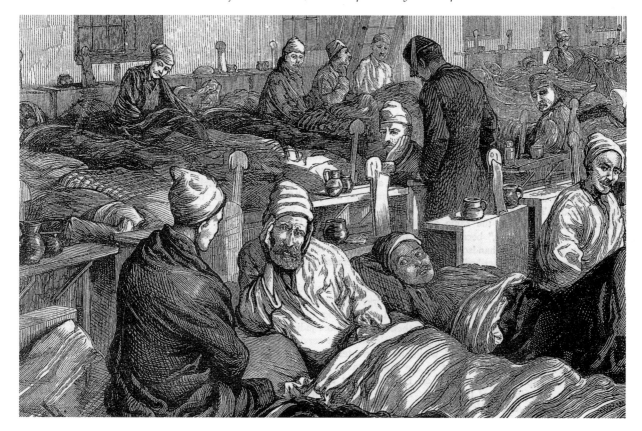

through activated charcoal, which absorbs the waste products. Another possible method is vacuum distillation followed by passing the vapor over a heated catalyst to burn off the organic contaminants. Recycling of urinary water is possible, then, although the idea cannot be considered especially aesthetic. However, our bodies also lose considerable amounts of water in sweat, through respiration and in the feces. Is there some method by which it could be collected and recycled?

In addition there is another problem concerning internal water and the possibility of living in space, namely the regulation of water balance in a weightless environment. On the earth when we stand up for a time, blood tends to pool in the legs through the effects of gravity. Lie down and this blood is displaced from the lower extremities, with the effect that a larger proportion of blood flows through the upper parts of the body. The outcome of this redistribution of blood flow means that

receptors in the large arteries emerging from the heart sense there is an apparent increase in blood volume. They switch off the release of antidiuretic hormone to try and compensate for this effect. In space, however, there is no pooling of blood due to gravity, and volume sensors continually inhibit antidiuretic hormone secretion. The result is diuresis, fluid loss through frequent urination or sweating. This may ultimately reduce blood volume so that the circulatory system is unable to respond to demands placed on it. (Actually, an even greater problem of living in a weightless environment is that of bone decalcification, a loss of calcium from the skeleton that makes the bones very fragile.)

It is simply not known to what extent the human body would be able to compensate or adjust to prolonged effects of weightlessness. But at all events, although human ability to adapt may not be the limiting consideration, what surely must be a decisive factor is the ultimate dependence of

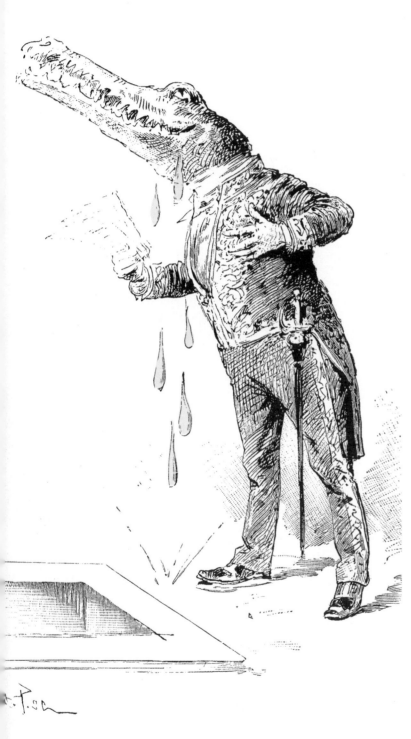

humans and indeed all living creatures on water for survival. Frank Herbert took up this question in *Dune*, his first book about the fictitious desert planet, parts of which in the deep desert are totally devoid of water. Other areas on the planet have only very small and precious amounts of this life-sustaining fluid. Herbert implies the physical adaptation of the inhabitants to their planet; their bodies apparently contain less water, and their muscles are consequently hard and relatively dry. He evidently recognizes the urgent need to conserve all the water that is possibly available, even to the extreme extent of recouping the water content of corpses.

The ultimate water-conserving devices that the author describes are the "Still Suits" which totally encompass the body of the Dune inhabitants. Tubes, valves, pumps and filtering systems, all intricately interconnected, enable any water lost from the body to be collected and recycled. This notion was conceived as science fiction, but in fact the technology exists to design and build a system to condense the water vapor in the air that is breathed out, and some sort of individual portable system for extracting water from urine. A mechanism for collecting the water lost in perspiration and sweat would be more difficult to construct, although creating a neutral and regulated microclimate within a space suit could negate the need to sweat and therefore restrict the amount of water lost from the skin. Maybe the most complex system would be one for recouping the water lost in the feces and disposing of only the solid waste material.

The sand worms in *Dune* may not have depended on water for their existence, but on earth water is the basic constituent for life, without which no living thing can survive. We take water for granted; it is always there to a greater or lesser extent, and much of the earth's surface is covered by great oceans, seas, lakes and rivers. Nevertheless, we are totally dependent upon our environment for our water needs, for although we have developed biological systems which help to conserve internal water, we continually need to replace the water we inevitably lose in urine, in sweat and in exhaled air. Without this regular replacement, survival time for a human being is short.

The successful conquest of space is largely constrained by the need for all living things to have a continuous supply of fresh water. With the impracticability of transporting water supplies from earth, one possibility is to recycle water lost through the skin, lungs and kidneys. An artist's impression of a space colony includes plant life and swimming pools, all contained within a huge rotating wheel.

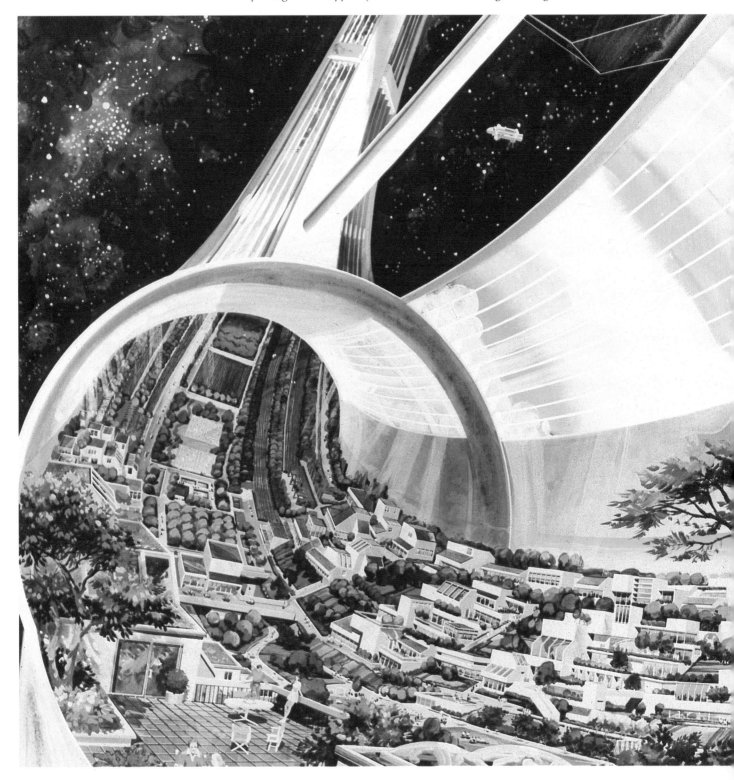

Glossary

ADH antidiuretic hormone.

adrenal gland an endocrine gland situated close above the kidney.

adrenal hormones hormones secreted by the adrenal gland. As well as some sex hormones and epinephrine (the fight and flight hormone), the adrenal hormones include corticosteroids, which are important in regulating salt balance.

albuminuria the condition of having the protein albumin in the urine.

aldosterone a hormone, produced by the cortex of the adrenal gland, which promotes the reabsorption of sodium.

amyloidosis a disorder in which amyloid, a waxy protein, forms and blocks blood vessels and kidneys.

analgesic nephropathy damage to the tubules of the kidney caused by a massive intake of painkillers.

anemia lack of hemoglobin in the blood.

antidiuretic hormone (ADH) a hormone from the pituitary gland that suppresses the flow of liquid into the urine.

antigens substances foreign to the body that stimulate the production of proteins to neutralize them.

anuria the cessation of urine production.

aorta the principal blood vessel by which blood leaves the heart to travel to the body.

aperient a drug with a purgative effect.

arterioles small arteries.

asepsis the use of sterilized equipment and conditions to exclude bacteria.

asymptomatic bacteriuria a condition in which significant numbers of bacteria can be found in the urine but without any symptoms of disease.

atherosclerosis thickening of the artery walls, with fatty or chalky deposits and fibrous tissue.

beta-blocking drugs drugs that weaken heartbeat and slow heartrate by inhibiting nerves to the heart.

biopsy the removal of a small piece of living tissue from the body for examination.

blood plasma the liquid part of the blood in which the blood cells are suspended.

blood urea nitrogen (BUN) the nitrogenous waste present in the blood as urea.

Bowman's capsule the dilated end of a kidney tubule surrounding a network of small blood vessels coming from the renal artery.

brush border the tiny projections from the surface of some types of cell in the gut and kidney, so-called because under the microscope they look like the tufts of a brush.

buffer a solution of salts in which the change in hydrogen ion concentration (pH) is minimal when an acid or alkali is added.

bulbo-urethral glands Cowper's glands.

BUN blood urea nitrogen.

calcium antagonists drugs used to lower blood pressure by reducing the amount of calcium entering the cells of the blood vessels.

calyces branches of the urine-collecting duct within the central part of the kidney.

cannula a small tube which is inserted into the body to withdraw or inject fluid.

CAPD continuous ambulatory peritoneal dialysis.

capillaries the tiniest blood vessels in the body.

capsule a membrane or coat around an organ.

cardiovascular of the heart and blood vessels.

casts small pieces of protein that have formed in the kidney tubules and have been washed into the urine.

catheter a tube inserted into a body cavity for the removal of fluid, especially of urine from the bladder.

cirrhosis a liver disorder in which fibrous tissue increases at the expense of liver cells.

coagulated of protein, solidified when subjected to heat; of blood, clotted.

continuous ambulatory peritoneal dialysis (CAPD) a type of dialysis in which the patient for most of the time is able to move around unconnected to any machine. Fluid, regularly changed, is put into the abdomen to extract waste, and the peritoneum itself is used as a dialyzing membrane.

corpuscles blood cells.

cortex the outer layer of an organ such as the kidney, adrenal gland or brain.

corticosteroids steroid hormones produced by the cortex of the adrenal gland.

Cowper's glands paired glands at the base of the penis secreting into the urethra.

creatinine a nitrogenous breakdown product of muscle which is filtered into urine.

Cushing's syndrome a disorder caused by a tumor of the pituitary gland, causing obesity, hairiness and other effects.

cystitis inflammation of the bladder.

cystoscope an instrument used to inspect the interior of the bladder.

detrusor the muscle layers of the bladder.

diabetes insipidus a disorder in which damage to the pituitary gland leads to the production of abnormally high amounts of dilute urine.

diabetes mellitus a disorder in which the pancreas does not produce sufficient insulin and large amounts of glucose appear in the blood and the urine. The urine volume is increased and the patient is thirsty.

dialysis   the separation of salts and other small molecules in solution from fluids containing these together with proteins and cells, by using a semipermeable membrane.

dialyzer   a machine to carry out dialysis.

diastolic blood pressure   the blood pressure at the time the heart is relaxing (rather than contracting).

diuresis   the production of urine, especially in quantity larger than normal.

diuretic   promoting the flow of urine, as do some drugs.

dropsy   edema.

dysplasia   an abnormality in development.

edema   the abnormal accumulation of fluid in the tissues of the body.

encysted   describes a microscopic organism which has secreted a protective capsule around itself and gone into a resting state.

end-stage renal failure   (ESRF) the situation in which a kidney loses all normal function.

endocrine system   the system of ductless glands and the hormones they secrete that control many of the body's activities.

endoscope   an instrument that can be inserted into a body cavity to allow viewing of its interior.

enuresis   involuntary passing of urine, as in bed-wetting.

epinephrine   a hormone produced by the medulla of the adrenal gland. Its effects prepare the body for "fight or flight."

erythropoietic factor   a substance produced by the kidney that stimulates the production of erythropoietin.

erythropoietin   a hormone that triggers production of red blood cells in the bone marrow.

ESRF   end-stage renal failure.

estrogen   the female sex hormone affecting sexual development and reproductive activity.

etiology   the causative factors of a disease.

excretion   emission from the body of the waste products of metabolism.

extracellular   outside the cell membranes.

fistula   an artificial pipe or passage created by surgery; a small fissure.

GFR   glomerular filtration rate.

globulins   a group of proteins found in many tissues, and soluble in dilute salt solutions.

glomerular filtration rate   (GFR) a measure of how well a kidney is functioning, the glomerular filtration rate is the amount of a substance cleared from the blood in one minute.

glomerulonephritis   inflammation of the kidney in which the glomeruli are mainly affected.

glomerulus   the network of small capillaries within a Bowman's capsule of the kidney, in which the primary filtration of the blood occurs.

gout   a disorder in which excess uric acid present in the blood is deposited at the joints, making them painful and sometimes deformed.

gouty tophi   hard crystal nodules of sodium biurate deposited in the tissues.

hematuria   the production of urine containing blood.

hemodialysis   dialysis of the blood in order to purify it.

hemoglobin   the red pigment of the red blood corpuscles that acts as an oxygen transporter for the body.

hemorrhage   the escape of blood from a blood vessel.

heparin   an anticoagulant, a substance which is able to prevent clotting of the blood.

hepatitis   inflammation of the liver.

hilus   the area of the kidney at which the main blood vessels and ureters pass into the organ.

histocompatibility antigens   proteins on the surface of cells that react against foreign cell material.

homeostasis   the maintenance of a constant internal environment by the body.

human chorionic gonadotropin   a hormone produced by the placenta that prevents degeneration of the corpus luteum in the ovary. This hormone passes into urine and its presence there is an indicator of pregnancy.

hydrocortisone   cortisol, an adrenal hormone sometimes used in the treatment of inflammation.

hypercalcemia   a condition in which the blood contains abnormally high amounts of calcium.

hypercalcuria   a condition in which abnormally high amounts of calcium are excreted in the urine.

hyperparathyroidism   a condition in which the parathyroid glands in the neck secrete more hormone than normal. This hormone raises the calcium level in the blood.

hypertension   blood pressure raised above the normal.

hyperuricemia   a condition in which the blood contains abnormally high amounts of uric acid, as in gout.

idiopathic   of disorders and conditions with no known origin, and apparently arising spontaneously.

immunosuppressive   describes a drug with the property of suppressing the body's natural immune reaction to foreign substances.

intermittent peritoneal dialysis   (IPD) a technique of dialysis in which a patient is from time to time coupled to a machine while dialysis takes place through the peritoneum.

internal meatus   the channel leading from the inside of the bladder to the urethra.

interstitial fluid the fluid surrounding and bathing the cells of the body.

intestinal flora the collection of bacteria normally present within the alimentary tract.

intracellular inside the cell or cells.

intravenous within, or put into, a vein.

involuntary muscle muscles such as those of the gut and arteries which act automatically rather than under the control of the conscious.

IPD intermittent peritoneal dialysis.

leukemia a type of cancer affecting the formation of white blood cells.

lipid-soluble soluble in fats and oils.

litholapaxy treatment that involves the breaking up of a bladder stone followed by washing out the fragments.

lithotomist one who practices lithotomy.

lithotomy surgical cutting into the bladder to remove a stone.

lithotrity the technique of crushing stones within the bladder.

loop of Henlé a loop of a kidney nephron that passes down into the medulla and back into the cortex. It allows reabsorption of some kidney filtrates.

lumen the cavity of an organ or duct.

lymphatic belonging to the lymphatic system, which drains the body tissues and returns fluid to the veins.

Malpighian body the glomerulus and its surrounding capsule.

medulla the central or mid-portion of an organ such as the kidney.

metabolism the chemical processes that take place within the cells of a living body, whether of building up or breaking down tissues.

metabolites substances produced as a result of metabolism.

microvilli the minute projections in a brush border.

micturition the passing of urine.

mitochondria the microscopic parts, or organelles, of a cell in which energy is produced.

mucous membrane a lining membrane well supplied with mucus ("slime") glands.

nephrology the study of the kidneys and excretion.

nephron one unit within the kidney, consisting of Malpighian corpuscle and its associated tubule.

nephrotic syndrome a kidney disorder in which there is edema and rapid loss of protein from the body.

nitrogenous waste waste products from protein breakdown, containing nitrogen.

nocturia a condition in which a patient has to urinate during the night with excessive frequency.

nonspecific urethritis (NSU) inflammation or irritation of the urethra; the cause may be obscure.

oliguria a condition in which abnormally small amounts of urine are passed and waste accumulates in the blood.

orchiectomy, or orchidectomy, the surgical removal of the testis.

osmolality the salt concentration of a solution.

osmosis the diffusion of a solvent through a semipermeable membrane from a weak to a strong solution.

osteomalacia a softening of the bone caused by the loss of calcium following vitamin D deficiency.

oxidation the "burning-up" of fats and carbohydrates in the course of metabolism, producing carbon dioxide and water.

pancreas a digestive gland, connected to the small intestine, which also includes tissue that produces the hormone insulin.

papillae the projections of the kidney medulla into the calyces of the urine-collecting duct.

papillary necrosis death of the kidney papillae.

paraplegic with the legs and lower part of the body paralyzed.

parathyroid glands four small hormone-secreting glands, close to the thyroid gland in the neck. The parathyroid hormone affects the level of calcium in the blood.

pediatrist a medical practitioner who specializes in childhood problems and diseases.

pelvic plexuses the networks of nerve fibers from which run the fibers supplying the cavity within the hip.

pelvis the hip region, particularly the hip bones; in the kidney, the cavity into which the tubules discharge urine, which is then drained by the ureter.

perineal in the region between the scrotum or vagina and the anus.

perirenal around the kidney.

peristalsis the involuntary waves of muscular contraction that push food through the gut, or urine along the ureters.

peritoneum a membrane which lines the abdominal cavity and extends across the viscera.

peritonitis inflammation of the peritoneum.

pheochromocytoma a tumor in the adrenal medulla, producing excess epinephrine and high blood pressure.

phosphocreatinine a compound in muscles which acts as a high-energy phosphate reservoir.

physiology the way in which a body or organ works, as opposed to its structure or anatomy.

pituitary gland an endocrine gland below the brain that secretes many hormones, including some that control the output of other glands in the body.

platelets small particles in the blood

that play a part in blood clotting.

polycythemia   thickening of the blood caused by an excess of red blood cells.

polyuria   excessive urine production with frequent urination.

progesterone   a hormone produced by the corpus luteum in the ovary.

prostate gland   a gland situated around the base of the urethra in males, and discharging into it.

prostatectomy   surgical removal of the prostate gland.

proteins   complex molecules built of long chains of amino acids, which are essential components of all living cells.

proteinuria   the presence of protein in the urine.

proximal tubule   the first part of a kidney tubule following the Bowman's capsule.

PTH   parathyroid hormone.

pyelonephritis   inflammation of the kidney and its pelvis.

radiotherapy   the treatment of a disorder such as cancer using radiation.

reflex   an action produced by a particular stimulus automatically, without conscious thought, mediated by a simple nerve pathway.

renal   of the kidney.

renal colic   a complaint in which there are severe spasmodic pains, usually caused by a stone lodged in the upper ureter.

renin   an enzyme produced from the walls of the blood vessels in the kidney which, acting through the intermediary angiotensin, affects blood pressure and urine flow.

reticulo-endothelial   a name applied to cells found in some connective tissue around organs, and lining some spaces in liver, spleen and bone marrow.

retroperitoneal   situated behind the peritoneum.

rickets   a condition involving soft and deformed bones found in children with vitamin D deficiency.

semipermeable membrane   a membrane that allows the passage of a solvent but not of large-molecule dissolved substances.

sensitized   a condition in which the immune system reacts with abnormal vigor to a foreign substance to which it has been exposed previously.

sphincter   a ring of muscle surrounding an orifice, closing it by contraction.

stenosis   the abnormal narrowing or constriction of a duct or vessel.

steroids   complex hydrocarbons, some of them natural hormones. Others are synthetic, but mimic hormonal effects or are used as therapeutic drugs.

stilbestrol   a synthetic estrogen.

stone   a hard concretion of mineral formed by disease within the body, known medically as a calculus.

suprapubic   above the pubic bone.

suprarenal   above the kidney. Suprarenal is an alternative word for adrenal.

testosterone   a male hormone produced by the testes which affects sexual development and reproductive activity.

tetany   a state in which the muscles are abnormally excitable and spasms occur.

thermoregulation   the processes involved in regulating the body temperature.

thrombosis   the formation, during life, of a clot within a blood vessel.

tissue typing   the categorization of tissue from individuals to determine the degree of compatibility with tissue from other individuals.

toxins   poisonous substances derived from living things, particularly poisonous substances made by microorganisms infecting the body.

transection   cutting through the long axis of a structure.

transfusion effect   the apparent link between having a blood transfusion and subsequent success of a transplant.

transitional cell carcinoma   cancer formed in the "transitional epithelium" of the bladder or ureter, a thin inner skin consisting of three or four layers of cells.

trauma   a wound or injury.

trigone   the area in the bladder, shaped like a triangle, between the two ureters and the urethra.

tuberculosis   a bacterial infection, usually attacking the lungs first, but spreading later, in which tubercles (or nodules) form in the body.

urea, or carbamide, a nitrogenous waste product, the chief organic substance in the urine of mammals.

uremia   a condition in which urea is retained in the blood instead of being filtered out.

ureters   the tubes, one from each kidney, along which urine passes to the bladder.

urethra   the duct by which urine passes from bladder to the exterior; in the male it also conveys semen.

urethral syndrome   discomfort in passing urine, for which a causative agent cannot be identified.

uric acid   a nitrogenous waste product of low solubility. It is used in birds and reptiles for excretion. In humans its presence in quantity causes gout.

urological   of the urinary tract, particularly its disorders, abnormalities, and their treatment.

vascular   of the blood vessels.

vasopressin   antidiuretic hormone.

vesical calculi   stones in the bladder.

vitamin D   a vitamin present in eggs, butter, fish livers and so on, that plays a vital part in maintaining the calcium balance of the body.

Illustration Credits

Introduction
6, Barnaby's Picture Library

The Water of Life
8, Martin Dohrn/Science Photo Library. 10, BP Chemicals. 11 left, Geoscience Features. 11 right, Brian Moser/ Camerapix Hutchison. 12 top, Wellcome Institute for the History of Medicine. 12 bottom, Geoscience Features. 13, *Salerno* by E. W. Cooke/ Guildhall Art Gallery, London/ Bridgeman Art Library. 14, Dr. Harold Rose/Science Photo Library. 15, BBC Hulton Picture Library. 16, Voigt/Zefa. 17, **Mick Saunders**. 18, Wellcome Institute for the History of Medicine. 19, Barnaby's Picture Library. 20, James Stevenson/Science Photo Library. 21, Wellcome Institute for the History of Medicine. 22, BBC Hulton Picture Library. 23, NASA/Science Photo Library. 24, M. I. Walker/Science Photo Library. 25, Nobelstiften, Sweden. 26, Hank Morgan/Science Photo Library. 27, Wellcome Institute for the History of Medicine. 28, University of Utah. 29, Dan Bernstein/Science Photo Library.

Fantastic Filters
30, Heilman/Zefa. 32, Melanie Friend/ Camerapix Hutchison. 33, Rod and Moira Borland/Survival Anglia. 34, **Mick Saunders**. 35, Bill Coward/ Barnaby's Picture Library. 36, **Mick Gillah**. 37, *The Pregnant Woman* by Raphael/Pitti Palace, Florence/ Bridgeman Art Library. 38, Barnaby's Picture Library. 39, Kobal Collection. 40, Scholz/Zefa. 41, Dieter and Mary Plage/Survival Anglia. 42, Al Giddings/ Survival Anglia. 43, **Mick Saunders**. 44, Glasshouse Crops Research Institute. 45, *The Public Bar* by John Henry Henshall/Christopher Wood Gallery, London/Bridgeman Art Library. 46, Mike Linley/Survival Anglia. 47, Tony Stone Associates. 48, *The Finding of Moses* by Sir Lawrence Alma-Tadema/Sotheby's, London/ Bridgeman Art Library. 49, Cavan McCarthy/Camerapix Hutchison. Foldout: Inner, Science Photo Library; **Mick Gillah; Mick Saunders; Norman Swift**. Outer, G. F. Gennaro/Science Photo Library. 50, United Artists/Kobal Collection. 51 top, Mary Evans Picture Library. 51 bottom, John Downman/ Camerapix Hutchison. 52, Tony Stone Associates. 53, Larry Mulvehill/Science Photo Library.

The Balancing Act
54, Biology Media/Science Photo Library. 56, Geoscience Features. 57, *The Baptism of Christ* by Piero Della Francesca/National Gallery, London.

58 top, **Mick Gillah**. 58 bottom, Camerapix Hutchison. 59, Mary Evans Picture Library. 60 top left, Rod Borland/Survival Anglia. 60 top right, Alan Root/Survival Anglia. 60 bottom, Camerapix Hutchison. 61, **Mick Gillah**. 62, Liesecke/Zefa. 63, **Mick Gillah**. 64, United Artists/Kobal Collection. 65, Zefa. 66 top, Steenmans/Zefa. 66 bottom, Zefa. 67, Kobal Collection. 68, Marion and Tony Morrison. 69, St Bartholomew's Hospital, London. 70, M. Saunders/ Camerapix Hutchison. 71, New York Heart Association. 72 top, Roger Viollet. 72 bottom, Ciba Geigy. 73, *Drug Store* by Edward Hopper/Museum of Fine Arts, Boston. 74, Mansell Collection. 75, Dr. Jeremy Burgess/ Science Photo Library. 76, M. I. Walker/Science Photo Library. 77 top, Camerapix Hutchison. 77 bottom, Sally and Richard Greenhill. 78, Camerapix Hutchison. 79, Michael Holford.

Diseases and Disorders
80, German Castro/Earthscan. 82, St Bartholomew's Hospital, London. 83, St Bartholomew's Hospital, London. 84, Sally and Richard Greenhill. 85, Everts/Zefa. 86, Barnaby's Picture Library. 87, Manfred Kage/Science Photo Library. 88, Geoscience Features. 89, Nobelstiften, Sweden. 90, Mary Evans Picture Library. 92, Michael Holford. 93, **Mick Gillah**. 94, St Bartholomew's Hospital, London. 95, Steenmans/Zefa. 96 left, St Bartholomew's Hospital, London. 96 right, St Bartholomew's Hospital, London. 97, **Mick Gillah**. 98, Moser/ Taylor/Camerapix Hutchison. 99, Sir Alexander Gibb and Partners. 100, **Mick Saunders**. 101, Camerapix Hutchison. 102, **Mick Saunders**. 103, St Bartholomew's Hospital, London. 104, St Bartholomew's Hospital, London. 105, Popperfoto. 106, Richmond Times. 107, Courtesy of the Trustees of the British Museum. 108, St Bartholomew's Hospital, London. 109, USDA.

Renal Replacement
110, Guy Gillette/Science Photo Library. 112, Popperfoto. 113, University of Utah. 114, **Mick Saunders**. 115, **Mick Saunders**. 116, North West Kidney Foundation. 117 left, **Mick Saunders**. 117 right, North West Kidney Foundation. 118 top, Russ Kinne/Science Photo Library. 118 bottom, Hank Morgan/Science Photo Library. 119, Larry Mulvehill/Science Photo Library. 120, Mary Evans Picture Library. 121, North West Kidney Foundation. 122, Shiley US. 123 top,

Shiley US. 123 bottom, Shiley US. 124, **Mick Saunders**. 125 top, North West Kidney Foundation. 125 bottom, Biophoto Associates. 126, North West Kidney Foundation. 127, Hank Morgan/Science Photo Library. 128, **Mick Saunders**. 129, Barnaby's Picture Library. 130, **Mick Saunders**. 131, Tony Stone Associates. 132, Hank Morgan/Science Photo Library. 133 top, Hank Morgan/Science Photo Library. 133 bottom, Hank Morgan/Science Photo Library. 134, MGM/Kobal Collection. 135, Will McIntyre/Science Photo Library. 136, Popperfoto. 137, Sandoz Pharmaceuticals. 138, Larry Mulvehill/Science Photo Library. 139, George M. Pantalos/University of Utah.

Environmental Influences
140, Schaeffer/Zefa. 142, Imitor. 143, **Mick Gillah**. 144 top, Baglin/Zefa. 144 bottom, Tony Stone Associates. 145, Tony Stone Associates. 146, Bromine and Chemicals Company. 147, *Water* by Guiseppe Arcimboldo/ Kunsthistorisches Museum, Vienna. 148 top, **Aziz Khan**. 148 bottom, St Bartholomew's Hospital, London. 149, **Aziz Khan**. 150 top, *A Halt in the Desert* by John Frederick Lewis/Victoria and Albert Museum, London/Bridgeman Art Library. 150 bottom, Jen and Des Bartlett/Survival Anglia. 151, Mary Evans Picture Library. 152, Mary Evans Picture Library. 153, NASA/Barnaby's Picture Library.

Index

cutting for, 16, 19, 20, **21**
  in mummies, **92**
  in the bladder, 16, **20**, 82
  in the kidney, 27, 28, 91, 93, **96**
  removal, 93, **97**
Streptococcus bacteria, 85
stress as a cause of infection, 88
stress incontinence, 38
stricture, urethral, 22
suprarenal gland, *see* adrenal gland
surgery, vascular, 25
sweat glands, primary function of, **11**
systemic lupus erythematosus, 105

T
temperature regulation, 56, 142
Tenckhoff catheter, 117
testosterone, 102
tetany, 72
thiazides, 77, 79
thirst, 60–61, 66, 76
  and seawater intake, 67
tissue rejection, 89, 130, **130, 131**
tissue-typing, **133**, 135, **135**
transferrin, 45
tuberculosis, renal, 91, **94**
  treatment of, 91
tubule, 11, 40, 42, 43, 141
  proximal, 43
tumor, hormone-secreting, 94
  of the urinary tract, 102, **103**
  Wilm's, 102, **104**

U
ultrasound as treatment for stones, 91
urea, 9, 13, **14**, 33, 47, 74
uremia, 21
ureter, 7, 9, 21, 34, **36, 55**, 78, 141
  contraction, 76
  damage to, 50
  nerve supply, 47
  triple, **83**
  twin, 36
    see also bladder

urethra, 7, 10, 19, 20, 22, 34, 37, 38, 77
  and urinary tract infection, 86
  blocked, 101
  damage to, 50
  prostatic, 37
urethritis, 88
  non-specific, 88
uric acid, **6**, 13, 33
  as a cause of gout, 105
  in birds, **35, 144**
  in the bloodstream, 28
urinary infection, 38
urinary space, 40
urinary tract, 21, 34
  infections, 86
  main organs of, **36**
  obstruction, 91
  tumors of, 102
urination, painful, 86, 88
urine, **6**, 10, 37, 38, 42, 51, 74, 100
  abnormal, 84
  and pregnancy testing, **72**
  as a bleach, **78**
  blood in, 13, 14, 31
  bubbles in, 38, **39**
  chemical composition of, 13
  coagulation, 13
  color, 12, 19, 86
  concentration, 43, **149**
  control, 103
  entering the bladder, **76**
  flow, 21, 101, **102**
  odor, 12
  penicillin extraction from, **75**
  production, 60, 66, 98
  regulation, 61
  retention, 14, 21, 101
  specimen, 86
  surface tension of, **39**
    see also incontinence
uroscope, 12
uroscopy, 12
  center for the study of, **13**

V
vaccines, 25

vasectomy, 22
vena cava, 35
  inferior, 42
venereal disease, 91
vesical sphincter, 37, 49
visceral cavity, 20
vitamin D, 72
  and rickets, 73
vividiffusion, 23
von Rosenstein, Rosen, 13

W
waste, 30, 112
  chemical, 30
  industrial, **80**
  metabolic, 33
  nitrogenous, 30, **35**, 45, 46, 142, **144**
  toxic, 21
water, 42, 145–149, **151**
  and Hindus, **70**
  and salt balance, 67, 143, 144,
    145–149
  control of, 60
  excess in the diet, **140**
  fountains of the Alhambra palace, 63
  lost as sweat, 34, 56, 146, 149
  lost from the lungs, 56
  lost in the urine, 33, 142
  percentage of body weight, **58**, 60
  reabsorption, 10, 11, 62, 142
  recycling in space, 151, **153**
  regulation, 33, 35
  retention, 85
  secretion, 11
  survival at sea, 145
  survival without, **65**, 143
  vapor, 34
White Lady spider, adaptation of, **60**
Wilm's tumor, 102, **104**

X
xanthine oxidase, 28
X ray, 82
  microdose system, **23**